A CRASH COURSE IN MODERN HEALTHCARE

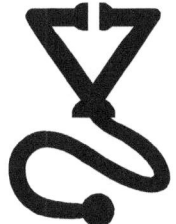

Published independently.

Copyright © 2024.

All rights reserved. No portion of this book may be reproduced in any form without permission from the authors, except as permitted by U.K. copyright law.

ISBN: 9798482295960.

Printed in the United Kingdom.

1st Edition.

A Crash Course in Modern Healthcare

Dr Matthew Williams

CONTENTS

About this book 7

Medical science 8
    Pathogens 9
    Zoonotic diseases 10
    Vaccines 11
    The immune system 12
    HIV 13
    Cancer biology 14
    Stem cells 15
    Antibiotic resistance 16
    Gut microbiota 17
    Structure and function 18
    Protein structure 19
    Action potentials 20
    Saltatory conduction 21
    Reflex Arcs 22
    Drug Development 23
    Drug kinetics 24
    Genome wide association study 25
    CRISPR/Cas9 26
    Laparoscopic surgery 27
    Dementia 28

Ethics & Law 29
    Pillars of medical ethics 30
    General Medical Council standards 31
    Mental Capacity Act 2005 32

- Mental Health Act 1983 33
- Medical paternalism vs patient autonomy 34
- The Montgomery case 35
- Ethics of euthanasia 36
- The Jehovah's witness blood transfusion dilemma 37
- Gillick competence and the Fraser guidelines 38
- Confidentiality and modern genetics 39
- HeLa cells 40
- Clinical Research ethics 41

Social Science 42
- Evidence based medicine 43
- Principles of statistics 44
- Measuring Disease burden 45
- Number needed to treat 46
- Sensitivity and specificity 47
- Positive and negative predictive values 48
- Survival Analysis 49
- Health inequalities 50
- Falls in the elderly 51
- Drugs on patent 52
- Technology in healthcare 53

Structure of the health service 54
- The formation of the NHS 55
- Primary, secondary and tertiary care 56
- Funding the NHS 57
- Distribution of NHS funds 58
- Allied health professionals 59
- Asylum seekers entitlement to NHS services 60

The medical career pathway 61
Applying to Medicine (UK) 62
Two-week wait pathway 63

History of medicine 64

Beaumont & St martin 65
Edward Jenner 66
Robert Liston 67
Ignaz SemmelWeis 68
John Snow 69
Aseptic technique 70
Marie Curie 71
The discovery of DNA 72
Thalidomide 73
PIP Breast implant scandal 74
The UK blood scandal 75
Alder Hey organ scandal 76
Bristol heart scandal 77
The MMR vaccine and autism 78
Theralizumab drug trial 79
Swine Flu pandemic 80
Novichok agents 81
Ebola 82
Severe acute respiratory syndrome coronavirus 2 83
COVID-19 84

ABOUT THIS BOOK

Modern healthcare is a fascinating and exciting field of work. Mankind's relentless and never-ending infatuation to cure disease and prolong life has culminated in an awe-inspiring array of evermore complex investigations, operations, and medical treatments.

Once, a simple laceration if infected would have been a slow and painful death sentence. Now, even the most gangrenous of wounds can be treated with a course of antibiotic. Not much over 200 years ago, an open long bone fracture would have necessitated an amputation where speed was the aim of the game and surgeons prided themselves on their stature, not just to wield the bonesaw but to simultaneously restrain the patient! Today, operations lasting 14 hours or more are feasible, with even the most essential anatomy temporarily bypassed, removed, transplanted, or even replaced with 3D printed replicas.

Healthcare has come a long way in the last 20 years, never mind the last 2000. What was once the idea of science fiction is now everyday practice and has changed or even saved the lives of millions. But innovation in healthcare has not come without sacrifice. The history of medicine is littered with stories of great tragedy and even scandal, all in the name of pushing the boundaries of medical practice.

Here we aim to tell the story of the sometimes dark and often controversial evolution of modern medicine. We guide you through: the delicate ethics and laws that underpin current practice, the essential scientific principles that dictate how our bodies function, the landmark historical discoveries of the common place techniques we use today, the complexities of social science that constrain the NHS, and finally the headlines and tragedies that have left medicine changed forever.

Whether you're a prospective medical student preparing for interview, a registered nurse looking for that band 6 position, or perhaps just someone with a morbid curiosity for the human body; we've sought to make this content applicable to all with each topic presented as a concise single page spread.

Individually interesting and an eclectic collection of fantastical stories, together they tell the story of how both landmark success and great tragedy have directed the evolution of medicine over the centuries, defined the role of the physician, and influenced the practice of modern medicine today.

MEDICAL SCIENCE

PATHOGENS

A pathogen is defined as an organism with the ability to cause a disease process in a host. The severity of that illness then describes that pathogen's virulence. Pathogenicity is conveyed by the production of toxins or cell surface receptors that permit intracellular invasion.

Pathogens span the full taxonomic tree from viruses to prokaryotic bacteria, to the vast array of eukaryotes both unicellular and multicellular including protozoa, fungi, and parasites. Not all pathogens are capable of causing disease in humans; there are approximately 1,400 known human pathogens.

> Prions are an increasingly recognised and terrifying pathogen. Misfolded proteins that cause host proteins to denature and bind together in large plaques. They are virtually indestructible, surviving standard hospital sterilisation techniques. They were found to be transmitting mad cow disease during bovine lens implants for cataracts and dementia between brain surgery patients from contaminated neurosurgical instruments!

It is estimated that over half of all humans that have ever lived were killed by a pathogen. Pathogens have therefore exerted a tremendous selective pressure in guiding our evolution and our history. For example, it was plague that decimated the city of Athens in 430BC and saved Sparta from certain defeat during the second year of the Peloponnesian war. And it was the measles and smallpox that they transmitted to the indigenous Aztec and Incan peoples that led the conquistadores to their sweeping conquests of the American colonies in the 16th century. The conquistadores in return contracted syphilis which later wreaked havoc throughout the royal courts of Europe.

Historically, pathogens occupied the majority of the physician's time. With advances in anti-microbial agents, immunisation, and an ageing population, there has been an epidemiological shift in the last 200 years. Smallpox that once riddled the UK has been eradicated thanks to Edward Jenner's discovery of vaccines. HIV can now be managed to undetectable levels with anti-retroviral therapy. The leading cause of human mortality is no longer infectious diseases but age-related processes like cancer, heart disease, and diabetes.

That said, with ready international travel and the diverse world in which we live it has never been easier for transmission of pathogens. The SARS outbreak in 2003, the recurrent Ebola crisis, the Zika virus in 2017, and more recently the COVID-19 pandemic in 2020 highlights the continuing burden of infectious diseases in modern medicine. Pathogens have shaped our history and will continue to guide our evolution.

ZOONOTIC DISEASES

PATHOGEN TRANSMISSION FROM ANIMALS TO HUMANS

Zoonotic diseases make up around 60% of existing infectious diseases in humans, and a greater proportion of emerging ones. This book discusses a number of them (Swine influenza page, Ebola virus, HIV, SARS-CoV-1 and -2, CJD), but other well-known zoonotic diseases include rabies, toxoplasma, and Lyme disease. Indeed, Jenner's first vaccine was to the virus causing cowpox, another zoonotic disease. Zoonotic pathogens can be bacterial, viral, parasitic, fungal, or prions (see page 13 about pathogens).

Zoonotic diseases can pass to humans directly from the natural reservoir or via an intermediate such as a tick or mosquito. Zoonotic pathogens sometimes have, or develop, the ability to also pass from human to human.

Historically, zoonotic diseases have increased in number and prevalence as humans have domesticated animals and increased their contact with them. There are concerns that climate change and environmental degradation are increasing the risks of zoonotic diseases as they push humans and animals into closer contact and diseases from warmer latitudes move north and south.

The change in geographic location of diseases is largely a result of vectors. Mosquitos carry and transmit malaria, dengue fever, Japanese encephalitis, and yellow fever among others.

> Avian influenza passes from birds to humans, but rarely causes human to human transmission. In 2012, controversial research was published showing just 5 specific mutations were needed to allow ferret to ferret airborne transmission. This caused concern surrounding a bioterrorism induced human pandemic given the ferrets are the best model of human influenza infection.

VACCINES

A SUBSTANCE THAT INDUCES IMMUNITY TO A DISEASE

Our immune system is exposed to external threats on a near constant basis. These threats are infectious diseases and present to the immune system as foreign antigens of a pathogen. For most threats (e.g. a strain of the common cold), a single exposure results in illness, then an immune system reaction that leads to elimination of the immediate threat (and thus recovery from illness), and prevention of this specific threat in the future.

However, in some instances the threat will evade our immune system, or the initial illness is so dangerous that we give vaccines to imitate infection and thus prepare our body for potential infection.

To imitate infection, vaccines must contain a substance that geometrically resembles an external part of a pathogen (the antigen). This can be dead or inactivated version of the whole pathogen, or fragments of it (sub-units). This elicits an immune response that subsequently destroys the vaccine, and then remains as immunological memory. If the pathogen subsequently enters the body and is encountered again, that same immune response eliminates the pathogen before infection can take hold.

Modern vaccines deliver the antigen along with an adjuvant. An adjuvant helps the body respond better to the antigen by inducing inflammation. Adjuvants stimulate dendritic cells of the immune system, which better mimics a natural infection and promotes better immune responses. Aluminium salt is a common adjuvant.

Smallpox is the first virus a vaccine was developed for. In 1796, Edward Jenner used cowpox to vaccinate against smallpox. Since then, the vaccine has been widely distributed, and smallpox was eradicated in 1980. Elimination of polio has almost been achieved via vaccination, and other diseases can be well controlled with vaccination. However, more complex pathogens such as HIV and malaria still pose huge challenges. This is largely due to the incredible variability of these pathogens.

This page has focussed on prophylactic vaccines that are used to prevent an infection. However, therapeutic vaccines that act to treat diseases once they are established are being developed. Notably, tumour antigens are being trialled for use in priming the immune system to destroy cancer cells.

THE IMMUNE SYSTEM

INNATE AND ADAPTIVE SYSTEMS

The innate and adaptive components of the immune system act in synchrony to protect humans from disease. At the crux of protection from disease is the ability to distinguish between self and non-self molecules.

When a pathogen enters the body, the innate immune system is the first line of defence. The innate immune system cells have ancient and highly conserved receptors (toll-like receptors) that recognise various non-specific pathogenic structures (e.g. double stranded RNA and bacterial flagellin) found on broad classes of pathogen. There are a number of cells in the innate immune system, but the classic group are known as 'phagocytes', cells which act to engulf pathogens and destroy them. Dendritic cells are a form of phagocyte that recycle the engulfed pathogen components and present them as antigens on their surface (earning the name 'antigen-presenting cell') for interaction with, and activation of, the adaptive immune system.

The adaptive immune system responds in a highly specific manner to each particular pathogen (or rather, the antigen associated with the pathogen), and there is immunological memory associated with this response. The adaptive immune response is facilitated by B cells and T cells and takes a few days to peak. The B cell arm of the adaptive immune system play a major role in antibody production, whereas the T cells are involved in direct killing of targets, such as cancer cells or virus infected cells.

> Severe combined immunodeficiency (SCID) is a genetic disorder in which there is aberrant development of both B and T cells. Patients often die in early childhood from overwhelming infections due to bacterial, viral, or fungal infections. David Vetter was born in 1971 with SCID as was referred to in the media as the 'boy in the bubble' as he lived in a sterile plastic chamber to protect him from pathogens. He lived until the age of 12, at which point he died after a bone marrow transplant he received had dormant Epstein-Barr virus, which reactivated and caused infection.

HIV

HUMAN IMMUNODEFICIENCY VIRUS

HIV is a virus with just 9 genes encoding only 19 proteins, yet it successfully invades the body, and then remains there indefinitely due to increasable powers of evasion. This evasion keeps it hidden not only from our immune system, but from anything that decades of intensive, and extremely expensive research have created.

The main targets of the HIV virus are CD4+ T cells, a type of white blood cell. This entry is mediated by the gp120 glycoproteins on the HIV viral envelope binding to the CD4 protein on the T cell. Once the virus is inside a cell, the host cell enzyme reverse transcriptase converts RNA into DNA. The 9 viral genes, now in the form of DNA, are then incorporated into the DNA of the host cell. These 9 DNA HIV genes are then encoded into RNA by the host cells transcription machinery. Some of this RNA is translated (again by host cell machinery) into the HIV proteins that assemble into new HIV viruses, whilst other RNA strands are packaged into these new virus structures. These HIV viruses that are contained within the CD4+ T cell then exit the cell to infect other cells.

HIV is incredibly adept at immune and drug evasion due to the rapid mutation rate of the HIV genome. This is in part due to the lack of proof reading after the action of the host reverse transcriptase. This mutation means the shape of the external glycoproteins (such as gp120) changes, meaning the immune system, and any vaccines we create, must play catch up. Integration of the HIV genome into the genome of the cells it infects means it is hard to clear the virus as all the cells that contain it must also be cleared from the body.

HIV infection has a brief period of flu-like illness, followed by an asymptomatic period that lasts months to decades. During this time CD4+ T cell levels drop until they reach such a low threshold that a person is diagnosed with AIDS (acquired immune deficiency syndrome). At this point the immune system is so damaged that people are at risk from many life-threatening infections.

CANCER BIOLOGY

SUSTAINED INDEFINITE PROLIFERATION OF CELLS

In health, the body has mechanisms for carefully controlling the number of cells in normal tissue. In cancer, non-lethal genetic damage causes individual cells to transition from healthy to cancerous. Cancer cells experience aberrant and sustained proliferative signals which result in the number of cells in a tissue increasing; the result is formation of a tumour.

Many different non-lethal genetic changes have been linked to cancer development, and any one cancer cell may have up to 100 different mutations.

These genetic changes can be linked to one of six basic 'hallmarks of cancer'. Each hallmark represents a distinct property that cells acquire. The hallmarks are as follows: self-sufficiency in cellular growth signals; insensitivity to cellular anti-growth signals, evasion of cellular death (apoptosis), unlimited ability to multiply (immortality), sustained angiogenesis signals, ability to invade tissue and metastasise. The need for such widespread changes is why cancer is relatively rare given the amount of cellular replication that the body undergoes in a lifetime.

Self-sufficiency in growth signals is analogous to an accelerator pedal being stuck down. There are mutations that mean an excessive amount of internal growth signals are produced by cells, which constantly stimulates them to grow and divide, forming a tumour.

Cells have a limit on the number of times they can replicate. This is the Hayflick limit and applies to differentiated cells (not stem cells). In healthy cells the Hayflick limit is about 50, which means that after around 50 cell divisions, a cell will be unable to divide again and is said to senescent. The reason for this is due to loss of telomeres (DNA at the end of each chromosome). Cancer cells avoid this if they have mutations that result in telomeres being protected or reformed.

> New cancer treatments are being developed that focus on inhibiting angiogenesis signals. This means preventing the creation of new blood vessels that is required to sustain tumour growth as cancerous cells grow and divide. This should help to slow the growth of tumours, and the Food and Drug Administration (FDA) in America has approved anti-angiogenesis strategies that are being used in conjunction with other anticancer chemotherapeutics.

STEM CELLS

CELLS FROM WHICH CELL LINES ORIGINATE

Stem cells are defined by their capacity to both self-renew and give rise to specialised cell types.

In mammals, during early embryonic development, a handful of embryonic stem cells (ESCs) are present. These differentiate and thus go onto form all the varying cell types found in the body. This ability to differentiate into any type of cell is a characteristic known as pluripotency. In order to maintain this population of stem cells and avoid them being 'used up' in differentiation, stem cells self-renew.

In adults, stem cells are found in a few places: bone marrow, fat, and blood. These are typically not pluripotent, meaning they can only differentiate into a subset of human tissue types.

Technology exists to allow differentiated adult cells to be reverted back to pluripotent stem cells. They are called induced pluripotent stem cells (iPSCs) and the discovery earnt the scientists responsible the 2012 Nobel prize. The Yamanaka Lab showed that addition of just four genes to somatic cells resulted in human fibroblasts transforming into induced pluripotent stem cells. The genes were Oct4, Sox2, Klf4, and cMyc and were delivered using a retroviral system. This technique has been refined and is now being applied to the field of regenerative medicine, and an area of excitement is iPSC-derived cardiomyocytes for use in future treatment of heart attacks.

> Stem cells as therapeutics: bone marrow transplant is a form of stem cell therapy that is well accepted. It is used for treatment of patients with bone or blood cancers who have had chemotherapy or radiotherapy to destroy their own immune system. Other more experimental treatments in regenerative medicine are being explored, many of which are involved in the treatment of ocular diseases. There is great promise around stem cells, but it remains to be seen how many research avenues make it to clinical practice.

ANTIBIOTIC RESISTANCE

AN EXISTENTIAL THREAT TO MEDICINE

Antibiotics are medicines that are used to treat bacterial infections. Bacteria are organisms that have a high replication rate, which allows genetic mutations to occur frequently. These mutations are occasionally advantageous for the bacteria, preventing them from being susceptible to antibiotics. Such bacteria survive and replicate, therefore leading to antibiotic resistance.

This is problematic in a clinical environment as it results in bacterial infections being harder to treat, leading to higher medical costs, prolonged hospital stays and increased mortality. Antibiotic resistance has increased over recent years due to these drugs being too freely prescribed for infections that do not require such treatment, as well as antibiotic courses not being finished.

Antibiotics target bacteria through several mechanisms. They can inhibit important enzymes involved in regulating the replication of bacteria, or interfere with cell membrane permeability and cell wall synthesis. They can also interrupt bacterial DNA and protein synthesis.

However, through advantageous mutations, bacteria have developed mechanisms to render them resistant to certain antibiotics. Bacteria can chemically inactivate antibiotics or alter the target site of the drug to reduce its binding capacity. They can also reduce the cell membrane's permeability to antibiotics or actively pump the drug out of the cell. The metabolic pathway that the antibiotic targets can also be altered, rendering the antibiotic ineffective.

The most problematic bacteria in hospitals is methicillin-resistant Staphylococcus aureus (MRSA) due to its resistance to a whole variety of antibiotics. MRSA epidemics are a huge threat to patients in hospital as these infections are so hard to treat. Only a handful of drugs are known that can effectively treat MRSA, such as vancomycin.

To combat the imminent threat of increasing antibiotic resistance, steps must be taken to prevent prescription of antibiotics for unnecessary infections as well as educating the general public about the importance of finishing full courses of the drugs. It is also important to consider the important effects of prophylactic prevention of infections through vaccinations, hand washing, good food hygiene and practising safe sex.

GUT MICROBIOTA

MICROORGANISMS OCCUPYING THE DIGESTIVE TRACT

It is commonly stated that humans are mostly microbes. This means the number of microorganisms found on or in our bodies (the majority of which are found in the gut) significantly outnumber human cells.

The microorganisms of the microbiota consist largely of bacteria (bacteriome). In addition, there are fungi (mycobiome), and bacteriophages (the main viral component of the virome). There is variation in the microbiota throughout the digestive tract, likely due to the pH gradient that begins in the stomach. Observable changes in the microbiota also occur after direct addition of bacteria (e.g. probiotics and faecal microbiota transplant) or after changes in diet (e.g. prebiotics, plant-based diets, high-fibre diets).

The presence of microorganisms in the human gut likely represents a mutualistic relationship, meaning there are benefits to both humans and microorganisms. Microorganisms benefit humans in a number of ways. They offer an alternative metabolic pathway to those provided by human enzymes. Some macro-fibrous material (colloquially known as fibre) requires bacterial enzymatic breakdown into short-chain fatty acids that can be used by host cells for energy. The microbiota also serves to defend against harmful bacteria, either by direct or indirect inhibition.

It has even been suggested that chemicals released by the gut microbiome can have far reaching effects on our metabolism and even our thoughts by travelling through the vagus nerve from our gut to our brains. Changes in the microbiota have been implicated to some degree in a number of chronic conditions e.g. type 2 diabetes, obesity, inflammatory bowel disease, and depression.

Faecal microbiota transplant (FMT) is revolutionising the management of patients with recurrent *Clostridium difficile* (*C. diff*) infection. *C. diff* is a bacterium that causes watery diarrhoea after colonisation of the colon, an event common after patients are treated with multiple classes of antibiotic (which have the side effect of killing aspects of the gut microbiota that normally keep *C. diff* in check). The principle of FMT is that microbiota from a health donor is used to reverse the bacterial imbalance in the affected patient.

STRUCTURE AND FUNCTION

THE LINK BETWEEN ANATOMY AND PHYSIOLOGY

Anatomy is the study of the structure of the body. Physiology, in its simplest form, is the study of the function of body. It has long been understood that the two are closely linked, as illustrated by the quote from Jean François Fernel, the 16th-century French physician: "Anatomy is to physiology as geography is to history; it describes the theatre of events."

There are many examples in the body to illustrate this integral relationship between structure and function; we will outline two examples related to tissue oxygenation, one from each of macro- and micro-scopic anatomy.

The heart has the dual function of pumping blood around the body, but also facilitating gas exchange at the lungs by maintain a concentration gradient for gases. As such, it is a double pump. It pumps high pressure blood that perfuses the tissues of the body, and lower pressure (thus slower moving) blood to the lungs to allow equilibration of gases. This is crucial in allowing effective gas exchange and delivery as a system with homogenous levels of pressure would be less efficient.

Red blood cells carry oxygen in the blood that diffuses into respiring tissues and as such have features that allow this to be optimised. The shape of the red blood cell is biconcave. This gives them a large surface are to volume ratio and allows them to fold into a bell shape and pass through tiny blood vessels with direct contact between the cell surface and the endothelial cells. The red blood cells have a flexible structural protein called spectrin. This allows them to fold and unfold many times as they repeatedly pass through capillary beds.

The red blood cell doesn't contain a nucleus or mitochondria, leaving more room for the haemoglobin that binds with Oxygen. Due to lacking mitochondria, red blood cells rely on anaerobic respiration. This also means they do not utilise any of the oxygen they are transporting, so they can deliver it all to the tissues.

PROTEIN STRUCTURE

PRIMARY, SECONDARY, TERTIARY, QUATERNARY

The order of amino acids that emerges secondary to the processes of cell transcription and then translation is the primary structure of proteins. Anfinsen's dogma stipulates that the resulting 3-dimensional protein structure is determined only by this primary structure.

The secondary structure of proteins is formed by the first stages of folding. Alpha helixes are stable helixes that are supported by hydrogen bonds that run in parallel with the helix, between every 4th peptide bond of the amino acid backbone. Beta-pleated sheets are a type of structure that forms the core of many proteins and have hydrogen bonds between discrete sections of the amino acid backbone that run parallel to each other. Chaperone proteins assist in this covalent folding, one crucial function of them is to prevent multiple polypeptide chains aggregating together erroneously.

The tertiary structure is the organisation of various elements of secondary structure into a defined 3-Dimensional shape. Covalent bonding in the form of disulphide bonds offer stability to the tertiary structure. In some proteins the assembly of multiple polypeptide chains gives a molecule its functional quaternary structure.

Even in a small polypeptide chain, there exists an incredible number of different possible conformations. Levinthal's paradox states that if a protein were to achieve its final shape by sequentially sampling each possible conformation, it would take longer than the age of the universe.

> Haemoglobin (Hb) and myoglobin (Mb) are oxygen carrying structures made of very similar polypeptide chains. The key difference is that Hb is made from 4 polypeptide chains, and therefore has a quaternary structure, whilst Mb has only one polypeptide chain. In Hb, the whole molecule changes shape as each polypeptide chain loads or unloads on oxygen molecule. As such the oxygen saturation curves of the two molecules are different.

ACTION POTENTIALS

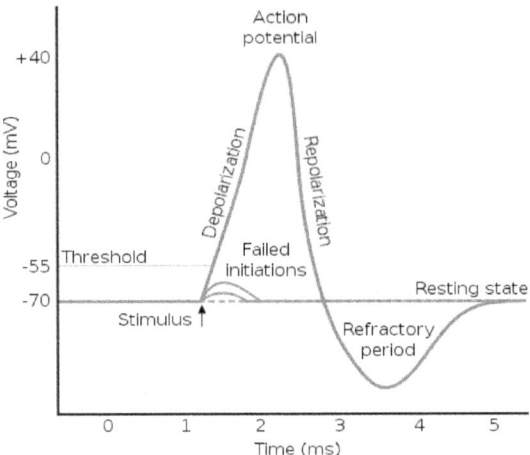

An action potential is an electrical signal that is transmitted via nerve cells. These allow different parts of the body to communicate.

To produce an action potential in a cell, a stimulus (such as pain, chemicals or temperature) acts on receptors to depolarise the cell. This stimulus must be large enough to depolarise the cell from −70mV to −55mV. If the stimulus is too weak, the initiation of the action potential fails. This is known as the 'all or none' principle.

The threshold voltage is reached when the cell depolarises to −55mV at which point voltage-gated sodium channels open resulting in a large influx of sodium into the cell. This depolarises the cell further to +40mV. The action potential is then fired either along the cell, or to a neighbouring cell to cause an effect.

The cell needs to then repolarise to allow for another action potential to be fired. At +40mV, the sodium channels close and potassium channels open, resulting in an efflux of potassium, which repolarises the cell. However, there is an overshoot as the cell repolarises past the resting membrane potential of −70mV.

The natural permeability of a cell allows restoration of the resting membrane potential. This is known as the refractory period and is necessary to allow further action potentials to occur.

SALTATORY CONDUCTION

Action potentials pass along nerves to transmit a signal from one area of the body to another (often involving the central nervous system). This involves a wave of depolarisation passing along the length of an axon. The depolarisation of one part of the axon as a result of an influx of sodium ions, triggers the activation of voltage gated sodium channels further along the axon. This leads to depolarisation in this area of the axon. Subsequent repolarisation via an efflux of potassium ions then occurs to ensure the next action potential can be conducted.

Nerve cells can be myelinated to allow the conduction of an action potential to be faster. This involves Schwann cells (in the peripheral nervous system) and oligodendrocytes (in the central nervous system) forming a myelin sheath around the nerve cell.

Myelinated nerve cells increase the action potential conduction velocity due to a process known as 'saltatory conduction'. Action potentials only occur at unmyelinated areas of the axon called nodes of Ranvier. The influx of sodium at these points causes the action potential to skip between the nodes via conduction of ions within the axon. This allows for electrical signals to be transmitted long distances at high rates without degradation of the signals. The conduction velocity of an action potential in a myelinated axon is roughly 150m/s compared to 2m/s in an unmyelinated axon.

> When the myelination around a nerve is destroyed the process of saltatory conduction is lost and this causes significant pathology. When a chronic progressive demyelination occurs in peripheral nerves Charcot Marie Tooth disease is the result, if it occurs in the central nervous system Multiple Sclerosis occurs. Alternatively, patients can present with an autoimmune destruction of their myelin sheaths, commonly after Streptococcal infection, and an ascending neuropathy in the form of Guillan-Barre Syndrome develops. This is generally self-limiting but sometimes mechanical ventilation can be required if the phrenic nerve to the diaphragm becomes involved.

REFLEX ARCS

A reflex arc is a neural pathway consisting of a series of nerves, a sensory cell and an effector cell. These are vital arcs that allow fast responses to particular stimuli. They tend not to involve the brain but synapse at the spinal cord to make them rapid reflexes.

A stimulus is sensed by receptors to trigger an action potential in a receptor cell. Stimuli can include temperature, pain or chemicals, which are sensed by thermoreceptors, nociceptors and chemoreceptors, respectively. A simple example is the withdrawal of a person's hand from a hot plate.

The stimulus (heat) activates the corresponding receptor (thermoreceptor) to depolarise the receptor cell, which, if large enough, will reach the threshold potential and fully depolarise the cell via voltage-gated sodium channels. This causes an action potential to be generated, which is transferred to a sensory nerve cell (neuron). The sensory neuron conducts the action potential to the spinal cord, where it synapses with a relay neuron. This relay neuron passes the action potential onto a motor neuron. The motor neuron conducts the action potential to an effector cell (a muscle cell or 'myocyte') at the origin of the signal. This causes contraction of the flexor muscles and subsequent withdrawal of the hand from the hot plate.

This whole process takes a very brief period of time, which is vital to ensure that tissues are not damaged by dangerous stimuli. The reflex arc is so fast because no processing by the brain is required, and the nerves involved are myelinated, so the signal is transmitted via saltatory conduction.

DRUG DEVELOPMENT

TRANSLATING SCIENCE TO THERAPEUTIC MEDICATION

Drug discovery is analogous to a rapidly narrowing pyramid. For each drug that is licenced, thousands of candidates that begin development are discarded.

Stage 1: Drug discovery. This begins in university laboratories where basic science allows for better understanding of disease processes. This may be the identification of a gene or protein that a treatment could interact with. A search then begins for a compound that matches this target. Historically this involved searching for natural compounds, however current technology allows for structural prediction of molecules that would be expected to have biological or pharmacological activity. Up to several thousand compounds are initially considered in this stage, which can take 5-10 years.

Stage 2: Pre-clinical trials. A few hundred potential compounds are tested *in vitro* in various models of the system they are designed for. If they remain candidates, they are also tested *in vivo* on animals. Toxicity, preliminary efficacy, and preliminary pharmacokinetics are studied.

Stage 3: Clinical trials. These are split into three phases, I, II and III. Only a handful of drugs make it to this stage, and only 10% of drugs that enter phase I clinical trials will ultimately gain FDA or MHRA approval. Phase I trials involve only a few dozen healthy human volunteers. These are mainly to evaluate tolerance and are carefully monitored. Drug pharmacokinetics are calculated in phase I, namely absorption, distribution, metabolism and excretion. Phase II involves a few hundred patients *with the disease of interest*. At this stage the drug is compared to a placebo treatment. Phase III involves a few thousand patients in randomised, multi-centre trials designed to definitively test the efficacy of the drug. Stage 3 takes 5-7 years and is typically extremely expensive. Following phase III, the drugs are submitted for consideration by the regulators, which in the UK are the Medicines and Healthcare Products Regulatory Agency (MHRA). Phase IV involves continued ongoing surveillance to detect any rare or long-term side effects.

> Google's DeepMind can now determine a protein's 3D shape from just its amino acid sequence. This is done using their AlphaFold tool and represents a stunning leap forward in structural biology that may have huge implications of the discovery of drug molecules.

DRUG KINETICS

ABSORPTION, DISTRIBUTION, METABOLISM, EXCRETION

Drug kinetics, also known as pharmacokinetics, describe how the body affects a substance after administration. The principles govern the amount of a substance that is present in a given part of the body at any time. The true currency of drug kinetics is equations and graphs, but we will illustrate the principles in a more accessible manner.

Whilst the application of a drug is not strictly involved in drug kinetics, a knowledge of the possible routes is useful. Possible routes of drug application, in rough order of time to effect, include; intravenous, inhalation, sublingual (under tongue), intramuscular, subcutaneous, rectal, oral ingestion. Topical (to the skin) application has a time-to-effect that his highly variable.

Absorption is the passage of a drug from the site of administration to blood in the vessels. With the exception of intravenous application, the rate of absorption differs depending on the route of administration, and the drug size, ionisation and lipid solubility (how easily it passes through the lipid component of biological membranes).

Upon entering the systemic circulation (blood), a substance distributes throughout the various compartments of the body (intravascular, interstitial, intracellular, and a few other smaller compartments such as the pericardium). Distribution reflects the physiochemical nature of the substance. It depends on permeability across tissue barriers, protein binding within compartments, and pH of the different compartments (differing pH's can change the properties of a substance).

The effect of drugs reduces due to metabolism and excretion. Metabolism is the biochemical changes that happen to a substance in the body. If a drug is given in its active form, metabolism will reduce its activity. In some instances, a pro-drug is given that is metabolised into an active drug in the body.

Drugs or drug metabolites are ultimately removed from the body by the kidneys, the liver, or lungs (for volatile or gaseous agent).

GENOME WIDE ASSOCIATION STUDY

CHARACTERISE PEOPLE BASED ON THEIR GENETICS

Underpinning the utility of genome wide association studies (GWAS) is the knowledge that genetic variation between individuals can cause altered observable characteristics (phenotype).

A GWAS starts with using high-throughput sequencing techniques to sequence the human genome.

A GWAS then looks at DNA sequence variations across the entire human genome to identify differences between healthy and diseased individuals. Genetic variants associated with a disease will be found at higher frequency in disease people than in healthy controls. These genetic variants typically take the form single-nucleotide polymorphisms (SNPs).

A GWAS allows us to identify who is at risk of a disease based on their genetics depending on the proportion of 'healthy' to 'unhealthy' SNPs they have.

We can also start to work out the biological mechanisms of disease so that new treatments can be developed. This is possible due to the central dogma of genetics in that genes affect mRNA which subsequently affects protein shape. However, this sort of analysis is best complemented by other forms of genetic investigation.

> GWAS can also be used to personalise medicine to a specific individual. For example, GWAS have helped identified a genetic variant that is associated with response to anti-hepatitis C virus treatment. The presence of absence of a specific SNP is associated with significantly altered response to the treatment. This finding, in combination with the ever decreasing cost of running a GWAS, has allowed doctors to make informed decisions about which treatment to give an individual patient. This approach to medicine will become more widespread as more basic science genetic research is translated into the clinical environment.

CRISPR/CAS9

GENE EDITING TECHNOLOGY

CRISPR/Cas9 makes up part of the immune system in prokaryotic organisms. It is a complex of two different structures, CRISPR and Cas. It provides a form of acquired immunity against foreign genetic material such as that present in viruses that infect bacteria (bacteriophages). It does this by breaking down this genetic material.

Natural immunity:

1. Sequence acquisition: Following an infection from foreign genetic material, a section of this is incorporated into the CRISPR structure.
2. Interference: Cas9 (CRISPR-Associated protein 9) is an endonuclease enzyme that cleaves the phosphodiester bond in a polynucleotide chain. CRISPR guides Cas9 to foreign genetic material that corresponds to that which is incorporated into CRISPR. Cleavage occurs and the threat from the foreign genetic material is nullified.

Genetic engineering:

> We have repurposed this system to allow the selective modification of genes in a cheap and reliable way. After identification of the sequence of genetic material that scientists want to modify (the site of interest), a section of this sequence is supplied to the CRISPR system. The CRISPR/Cas9 is then delivered into the cell of interest. The CRISPR and associated genetic material guides the Cas9 enzyme to the site of interest, where it cleaves the DNA.

At this point there is flexibility in what can happen next:

- A double strand break induces DNA repair pathways that are prone to error, and this can disrupt the gene, and resulting protein.
- Providing a DNA repair template with the CRISPR/Cas9 allows for the insertion of a specific sequence at the site of interest.

LAPAROSCOPIC SURGERY

A 20th CENTURY SURGICAL INNOVATION

Laparoscopic, or "keyhole", surgery is a form of minimally invasive surgery which utilises a telescopic video camera (or laparoscope) to visualise the abdominal and/or pelvic viscera without the need for large open incisions.

The most well-known example of this mode of operating is the laparoscopic cholecystectomy (a keyhole gallbladder removal) where the traditional Kocher approach (a 15cm incision running parallel to the border of the right ribs) is replaced with 3-4, 5-10mm, ports with the gallbladder finally removed through a port adjacent to the umbilicus.

The concept evolved back in 1910 from Kelling's work in dogs before Jacobaeus applied the technique to humans later that year. In a time before video cameras and television screens Jacobaeus peered down the eye piece of a modified cystoscope (normally used to see inside the bladder) to diagnose tubercular adhesions.

The use of laparoscopy remained solely diagnostic for many decades since many surgeons had reservations about the difficulty in controlling a bleed with such minimal access. From the 1940s, much of the innovation surrounding keyhole surgery was driven by Palmer, a gynaecological surgeon, who used the technique to perform tubal ligation procedures. As the techniques and technology continued to develop, general surgeons began to take interest and in 1985 the first laparoscopic cholecystectomy was performed by Mühe in Germany.

Laparoscopic surgery has many benefits: less invasive procedures, smaller scars, quicker recovery times resulting in shorter hospital stays and reduced rates of post operative complications. It is important to remember that not all operations have been improved by the use of keyhole techniques. For example, it has been widely proven that carpal tunnel decompression shows superior outcomes when performed using traditional open procedures as all the relevant anatomy can be readily visualised.

> The idea of minimally invasive surgery continues to evolve. Cardiothoracic surgeons now use thoracoscopes to see inside the chest and orthopaedic surgeons can operate within joints arthroscopically. A 21st century adjunct is the use of robots which can even operate through a single 10mm incision or remotely. In 2001, the Lindbergh operation saw a group of French surgeons based in New York perform a robotic laparoscopic cholecystectomy on a patient in Strasbourg thousands of miles away!

DEMENTIA

NOT AN INEVITABLE CONSEQUENCE OF OLDER AGE

Dementia refers not to one disease in particular, but rather a syndrome of symptoms that can have a number of different underlying causes. Dementia describes a loss of memory, language, and critical thinking which is severe enough to interfere with daily living. It is a chronic condition for which there is currently no cure.

There are approximately 55 million people living with dementia worldwide with a further 10 million new diagnoses each year. According to the World Health Organisation this makes dementia the seventh most common cause of death in the world and a leading cause of disability.

Dementia is often incorrectly assumed to be a disease of older age or even part of the normal ageing process. This is not the case. Many older people will live a full and independent life, and whilst they may become more forgetful as they get older this does not significantly interfere with day-to-day living, and therefore does not constitute a diagnosis of dementia. Dementia represents cognitive decline beyond what is expected of normal biological ageing.

Frequently the terms dementia and Alzheimer's disease are used interchangeable. They are, in fact, not one and the same. Whilst Alzheimer's disease is indeed the leading cause of the dementia syndrome (estimated to represent some 60 – 70% of cases), it is not the only one.

Other aetiologies include:

- Vascular dementia - the result of disrupted blood supply to the brain.
- Frontotemporal dementia – this tends to affect younger adults from the age of 45.
- Lewy body dementia - caused by a similar pathology to that of Parkinson's disease.

A strict diagnostic work up is required for a diagnosis of dementia, including a full history and examination, blood tests, brain imaging, and specialist follow up in secondary care (a hospital memory clinic). This can take some time which is often frustrating for family. Whilst a formal diagnoses of dementia changes very little from a treatment point of view, it does enable access to specialist services which focus on social care to safely manage the symptoms of dementia.

ETHICS & LAW

PILLARS OF MEDICAL ETHICS

THE BASIS OF APPROACHES TO MEDICAL ETHICS

AUTONOMY

Doctors must allow patients to make their own decisions. It is the responsibility of the doctor to convey all the necessary information in an impartial way at a level the patient can understand. Following this, every patient has the right to make a 'bad decision' (from the perspective of the doctor) if they have capacity (see page 36 for more on capacity).

BENEFICENCE

To be caring is an important quality for a doctor, since beneficence refers to promoting what is best for the patient. The most obvious example of this is prescribing pain relief. An important consideration is that beneficence sometimes requires doing nothing when the benefits of treatment are minimal and the risks high.

NON-MALEFICENCE

This is the principle of do no harm. Whilst on the face of it this may seem obvious, it is important to remember that many treatments (drugs or operations) carry the risk of potentially harmful side effects or complications. As such the combination of beneficence and non-maleficence requires clinical skill, and calls for a careful balance of risk and benefit to the patient.

JUSTICE

As a doctor you will treat many thousands of patients throughout your career and indeed many thousands are treated in the NHS each and every day. However, resources are limited and not everyone can be cured. Justice refers to the rightful allocation of resources where they are needed and where they can be most beneficial. It is from this that the principle of triage emerges.

GENERAL MEDICAL COUNCIL STANDARDS

PROFESSIONAL STANDARDS AND MEDICAL ETHICS

The General Medical Council (GMC) regulates doctors in the UK with the aim of protecting the safety of the public.

The GMC maintains a register of medical practitioners, all of whom are required to revalidate on a regular basis. The GMC also investigates any concerns that arise about a doctor's fitness to practise and if necessary, they remove a doctor from the register (this is when a doctor is said to be "struck off").

The GMC sets professional and ethical standards for doctors to adhere to. The bulk of guidance is published in a document called 'Good Medical Practise' although more specialised topics such as confidentiality, end-of-life care, and prescribing have their own documents.

Good Medical Practise describes what it means to be a good doctor. It states that a good doctor will:

- Make the care of their patient their first concern.
- Be competent and keep their professional knowledge and skills up to date.
- Take prompt action if they think patient safety is being compromised.
- Establish and maintain good partnerships with their patients and colleagues.
- Maintain trust in them and the profession by being open, honest and acting with integrity.

The GMC offer guidance for medical students and expect them to demonstrate behaviour in keeping with their place as future members of the medical profession.

MENTAL CAPACITY ACT 2005

A LEGAL FRAMEWORK FOR ADULTS LACKING CAPACITY

Capacity refers to a patient's ability to understand and use information to make their own decisions about their care. There are a whole variety of reasons why a patient may be unable to make a decision. A patient is said to lack capacity to make decisions if their normal thinking is impaired in some way. In older adults it is often as a result of neurodegenerative diseases such as dementia. It is crucial to note that all adults are presumed to have capacity unless proven otherwise.

A patient's capacity can vary over time and so it must be assessed on a situational basis. For example, a patient with advanced dementia may well possess the capacity to decide what they would like to eat for dinner, but it is unlikely they would have the capacity to consent to a complex surgical procedure for which there is a large amount of information to be reasoned.

A formal capacity assessment is carried out by a trained healthcare professional in line with the Mental Capacity Act, and focusses on four main questions:

1. Can the patient receive and understand information?
2. Can the patient retain this information?
3. Can the patient weigh up the information to reach their own decision?
4. Can the patient communicate this decision?

If the answer to any of these questions is no, then the patient is said to lack capacity. In this instance every effort must be made to provide the minimum care necessary for the patient to regain capacity.

In the event that a patient does not regain capacity then doctors are bound by a strict legal framework (the Mental Capacity Act). The patient may have an advanced directive in place such as a "do not attempt CPR" order. Alternatively, the patient may have appointed power of attorney to a close relative. Both of these are legally binding decisions that the patient can make at a time when they are deemed to have capacity. If neither of these options are present, then doctors are expected to act "in the patient's best interests" with the least restrictive intervention.

MENTAL HEALTH ACT 1983

A LEGAL FRAMEWORK FOR DETAINING PATIENTS WITH MENTAL HEALTH ILLNESSES

The Mental Health Act (1983) is a set of laws that covers the assessment, treatment and rights of people with a mental health disorder. The majority of patients treated in clinical setting have agreed to their treatment. However, under the Mental Health Act, a patient can be treated involuntarily. This process is called 'sectioning' and can be done if a patient has a mental disorder that puts them, or others, at risk.

There are different sections of the Mental Health Act, and each specifies a different situation in which a person can be detained. These vary in many ways such as the length that they can detain a patient for, the treatment that is allowed to be given under such a section, and the medical staff able to apply the section.

These are some of the key sections to be aware of:

Section 2: This allows a patient to be detained for 28 days for assessment. It must be applied by an approved mental health professional (AMHP) and recommended by at least two doctors.

Section 3: This is similar to Section 2 but it is an admission for treatment rather than assessment and therefore can last up to 6 months.

Section 5(2): Allows a doctor to detain a patient who is already admitted to hospital, with an emergency holding order, lasting up to 72 hours. They are then assessed within this time before a plan is formulated.

Section 5(4): This is similar to the Section 5(2) but is used by a nurse to detain a patient for up to 6 hours.

Section 136: This allows police to remove a person, who is potentially at risk of harming themselves or others, from a public place and convey them to a place of safety for up to 72 hours.

Section 135: This is like a Section 136, but the person is located in private accommodation rather than a public place.

MEDICAL PATERNALISM VS PATIENT AUTONOMY

EVOLUTION OF THE DOCTOR PATIENT RELATIONSHIP

As you will have read on page 34, autonomy is one of the ethical pillars supporting good patient centred care. Despite this, throughout much of history, certainly up until the early 20th century, medicine had adopted a paternalistic approach at the expense of the patient's autonomy.

Medical paternalism sees the physician assuming to take ownership over the patient's welfare, making core decisions regarding their care often without consulting the patient. With an almost god-like presence physicians were seen to always act in the patient's best interests, owing to their expertise and medical training, with the patient expected to dutifully comply without question.

Needless to say, this hierarchical dynamic is not conducive to a healthy doctor-patient relationship. In recent decades medicine has entered a new era of patient autonomy. This has largely been driven by the explosion of the internet and social media providing easy access to medical information which has empowered patients to be less reliant on physicians.

This concept of "Dr Google" has of course reared its head in the news over the years exemplifying a recurring theme in medicine, which is that book smart knowledge is often not superior to on the ground experience. Nevertheless, patients increasingly arrive for their consultation having thoroughly researched their symptoms and identified possible diagnoses, and those with rarer chronic conditions may indeed be more knowledgeable about their condition than the doctor.

In a new era of patient centred care, the doctor's role is to support and enhance this patient autonomy rather than combat it through archaic medical paternalism. One could argue the roots of the word "doctor" (derived from the Latin for teacher) are more pertinent than ever as the modern idea of informed consent now sees physicians providing patients with the relevant information and options to make their own decisions regarding their care.

THE MONTGOMERY CASE

A NEW PRECEDENT IN MEDICAL CONSENT

In this legal case, Nadine Montgomery, a patient with diabetes, was expecting the birth of a large baby boy (this is a known complication of diabetes in pregnancy). She proceeded with a natural vaginal birth as advised by her obstetrician. During the delivery her son suffered shoulder dystocia with subsequent hypoxic insult of his brain causing cerebral palsy.

Montgomery claimed that her obstetrician failed to disclose any of these events as potential risks of a diabetic vaginal birth, even when she directly queried the baby's size herself. She sued for clinical negligence, claiming that should she have been made aware of the potential dangers she would have elected for a caesarean section. In March 2015, the UK Supreme Court ruled a landmark victory in Montgomery's favour, setting a new precedent for informed patient consent.

This ruling invalidated the incumbent legal precedent. This was the "Bolam test" which had been used to assess clinical negligence in previous cases. The Bolam test determined quite simply whether the actions of the accused would have been replicated by an independent body of medical professionals – note the lack of any input from the patient. The Montgomery ruling therefore demonstrated the need for patient involvement in clinical decision making. A patient must be made aware of any 'material risks' involved in a proposed treatment, and of reasonable alternatives.

The test of materiality in any particular case is whether "a reasonable person in the patient's position would be likely to attach significance to the risk, or the doctor is or should reasonably be aware that the particular patient would be likely to attach significance to it."

This was a significant event in redefining the role of the medical professional in the modern patient-doctor relationship in terms of the law. Marking a clear transition from medical paternalism to the autonomous patient.

In the modern era of patient centred care there is increased emphasis on the dialogue between patient and doctor, and particularly the facilitation of informed consent. In a "good" consultation, the doctor will try to ascertain what is important to the patient such as hobbies, lifestyle etc. This allows the doctor to present relevant information to the patient in a way that they can understand and process to arrive at their own informed decisions. This is the fundamental outcome of the Montgomery ruling.

ETHICS OF EUTHANASIA

DELIBERATELY ENDING A LIFE TO RELIEVE SUFFERING

Euthanasia is when an individual takes action to end another's life, with the sole motivation being the best in the best interests of the person who dies. Euthanasia encompasses differing doctor's actions (active vs passive euthanasia), and differing patient involvement (voluntary, non-voluntary, and involuntary euthanasia, the latter of which is illegal and opposed in almost all circumstances). Other associated ideas include assisted suicide, and principle of double effect.

In the UK, active euthanasia is when an individual takes direct action to end another's life. This is regarded as murder and treated as such in the courts. Assisted suicide, for example obtaining but not administering life-ending drugs, is also illegal in the UK, however this is legal in Switzerland and there is reasonable knowledge of this in the general population. Passive euthanasia, the removal of treatment required to sustain life, is not illegal in the UK.

The principle of double effect is a mechanism via which it is permissible to relieve a patient's pain, even if a foreseeable consequence is shortening of life. An example of this is the use of opioid drugs. These drugs, such as morphine, as powerful analgesics, but also potent respiratory depressants.

Euthanasia can be approached with the framework of the four pillars of ethics. Those in favour state that a person should have autonomous choice over how they die, and that with beneficence and non-maleficence in mind, doctors should aim to minimise the suffering of patients. Those against state that to prematurely end a life to cause harm, and this violates the principle of non-maleficence.

> Dr Cox was a rheumatologist who administered potassium chloride (KCl) to a well-known patient of his who was in extreme pain at the end of her life. This was said to shorten her life by less than an hour and qualifies as active euthanasia. The patient's family thanked Dr Cox. Dr Cox was charged with attempted murder. He was given a 12 month suspended sentence, and no further action was taken by the GMC and Dr Cox returned to his job.

THE JEHOVAH'S WITNESS BLOOD TRANSFUSION DILEMMA

This classic medical school interview questions requires a number of ethical and legal principles to be considered and can present in many situations.

The first, and potentially simplest situation, is that of a parent refusing on behalf of their unwell child. Whilst parental consent is normally required to perform any procedure on a child, parents are not permitted to make decisions that may harm the child. There is therefore no legal debate to support the parent blocking the child's blood transfusion. Clinicians are entitled to proceed in the child's best interests, seeking a court order if needed (hospitals will have lawyers on call 24 hours a day for this sort of situation).

A similar situation, considering an adolescent patient, is not as clear cut legally but ultimately ends with the same result. Gillick competence, see overleaf, means that older children who are able to understand the risks and benefits regarding a procedure can consent to (but not refuse) it irrespective of their parent's opinion. If, however, both parent and adolescent patient refuse consent to treatment then as above, the patient is a minor, and the clinician proceeds with a best interests decision to treat.

How does this situation pan out in the adult patient? Well, recall from page 36, any patient with capacity, acting autonomously and informed of all the relevant risks has the right to refuse treatment with or without a valid reason. But what if, for example, the patient is unconscious as a result of a serious road traffic collision, and therefore lacks capacity? A relative tells you of the patient's religious beliefs and you find a signed blood product refusal card in their pocket – do you still withhold lifesaving treatment?

Well as per our earlier discussion on capacity, when a patient is incapacitated, the clinician can look to an advanced directive (the refusal card) or act in the patient's best interests (drawing on the relative's knowledge of the patient's beliefs). However, the clinician is not to know whether the advanced directive was signed under coercion or even if the patient still holds that view since it was signed. Similarly, it is not beyond the realms of possibility that the patient had described false beliefs to their relative for fear of judgement or persecution. The point is, in the heat of the moment, it is not appropriate to assume second hand information at face value. The doctor is well within their rights, as per the mental capacity act, to provide the minimum treatment necessary, in best interests, for the patient to regain capacity and therefore make their own decisions surrounding their care.

GILLICK COMPETENCE AND THE FRASER GUIDELINES

The principle of Gillick competence allows young adults, under the age of 16, to consent to treatment without parental input if they demonstrate appropriate maturity and understanding.

The idea stems from legal proceedings that started in 1982, when Victoria Gillick took the West Norfolk and Wisbech Area Health Authority to court, in an attempt to block doctors giving contraception to under 16s without parental consent. In 1984 the case was presented before the High Court. Gillick's claims were dismissed. This decision was temporarily reversed by the Court of Appeals later the same year before, in 1985, the case was taken before the House of Lords who ruled in favour of the initial verdict and Gillick's claims dismissed once more.

This outcome has set a legal precedent in the UK that is not infrequently applied by doctors. It remains a controversial idea, because not only does it allow patients under the age of 16 to seek medical treatment without input from their parents, but it allows them to proceed with care against their parent's wishes if deemed in their best interests. It is important to note that Gillick competence only permits the consent to specific treatments offered by a physician and it does not empower minors to refuse medical treatment if it could lead to harm.

A special application of the principles of Gillick competence is seen in the Fraser guidelines, which specifically refer to advice and treatment for under 16s regarding contraception and sexual health, including treatment of sexually transmitted infections (STIs) and abortion. The Fraser guidelines provide legal backing for healthcare professionals to offer treatments in the patient's best interests if: they cannot be persuaded to inform their parent/guardian, the young person understands the risks and benefits involved, there is no coercion or pressure, and the young person is likely to continue having sex with or without contraception.

There is a fine line to be tread between empowering young adults and identifying significant child protection issues. Underage sex remains a significant identifier of child exploitation. As such there are several caveats to the Fraser guidelines which always result in child protection referrals, most notably minors younger than 13 (the age below which sex is always statutory rape) seeking contraception, and frequent presentations for the treatment of STIs and/or abortions.

CONFIDENTIALITY AND MODERN GENETICS

TECHNOLOGY IS FORCING A RE-THINK OF STANDARDS

Inherent to undertaking genetic testing and diagnosing a hereditary condition is the consequence of discovering information about the relatives of the patient. This differentiates genetic testing from most other forms of medical testing where the information is only relevant to the patient, and therefore decisions about confidentiality are more straight-forward.

A doctor has a duty to protect confidentiality and also a duty of care. As outlined by the GMC, there are certain circumstances whereby it may be appropriate to break confidentiality.

One such circumstance is the revelation of a genetic diagnosis that likely affects a family member. Ideally, the patient will consent for sharing of information, but in some cases they will not. Resolution of conflicts in these situations will inevitably require subtlety rather than adherence to rigid guidelines and medical practitioners must undertake a balancing act and must properly consider the implication of this and their duties.

> ABC v St Georges Healthcare and Others [2020]: this is a complex case that is worth reading in more detail. It relates to confidentiality surrounding a Huntington's disease diagnosis in a father, and the accidental disclosure of this to a daughter who was at the time pregnant. The daughter contended that the team caring for her father ought to have informed of her risk in time to be able to choose to terminate her pregnancy, even though her father had explicitly not consented to this.

HELA CELLS

A CELL LINE USED EXTENSIVELY IN RESEARCH

Henrietta Lacks (1920-1951) was a patient at Johns Hopkins hospital in Baltimore who was being treated for cervical cancer.

The eponymous HeLa cells are derived from those taken from one of Henrietta Lacks' tumours on the 8th February 1951. These cells were cultured and were found to be 'immortal'. In a cellular sense this means they do not die after a finite number of cell divisions (a defining property of cancer). Prior to the HeLa cells, any other cells cultured from human cells survived for a few days at best.

This discovery represented a significant improvement in medical research capabilities. Experiments involving cells could then be repeated on exactly the same batch of cells, and the effort to sample and culture cells reduced enormously. As such, demand for HeLa cells quickly increased. Notably they were used in the development of the Polio vaccine in 1952, and today are still widely used to test chemotherapy drugs. Research using HeLa cells has been published in many tens of thousands of scientific papers. A number of ethical issues surround the cells:

- Informed consent was not given by Henrietta Lacks, nor any of her family. In fact, it was not until two decades after initial culture that the family learned of the existence of the cells.
- In 2013, the complete genome of the HeLa line was sequenced and published online without family consent. At the time this broke no rules or laws but was ethically dubious. This intensified criticism about the privacy of the Lacks family. In response, the data was removed from public access and new legislation was put in place to ensure that applications to study it must be reviewed by a committee including members of the Lacks family.

> Poliomyelitis (polio) is an infectious disease that is symptomless in around 75% of those infected. However, a small proportion get paralytic poliomyelitis, and this made the disease devastating. The first effective polio vaccine was developed by Jonas Salk in 1952. Salk's vaccine was a dead-virus injectable vaccine. The HeLa cells were crucial for developing the vaccine as the cells could be infected by the virus yet still survive, hence allowing research to be conducted.

CLINICAL RESEARCH ETHICS

PRINCIPLES BASED ON THE FOUR PILLARS

Research is the process by which knowledge is produced and therefore medical care improved. Clinical research relates to clinical trials of new drugs or interventions.

In clinical work, ethical conflicts lie in determining what constitutes acting in the 'best interests' of a patient. In contrast, in clinical research the ethical conflict involves balancing the interests of the patient against those of medical science.

When patients get involved in clinical research they may benefit, they may have a neutral experience, or they may be harmed as a direct consequence of being involved. Research is a crucial step in the progression of medical care, and so society derives benefit from it. Nonetheless, it is crucial to ensure that exposing individuals to the risks of research is worth it for the sake of others; this is what research ethics approval is about.

At the crux of ethical research is informed consent. Each participant should have capacity to make the decision, should be fully informed about the research, and they should take part voluntarily.

To be fully informed about participation in clinical research means that a person understands the research. For example, they understand the research aims and methods, the risk of receiving the control treatment, the discomfort and inconvenience involved, their right to choose not to be involved or to withdraw at any time, and the fact that this will not change any other aspect of their care.

Consideration must also be given to the fact that even if there is informed consent, it still may be unethical to undertake the research if the risks are too great.

> Given informed consent is a necessary condition for research participation, those with life-threatening illness that limits capacity should be considered ineligible. However, if this were the case, we would have no emergency medicine research, for instance into the effectiveness of adrenaline in cardiac arrests. The way this is dealt with is via well publicised opt-out options, and consent by proxy by family members. The ethical considerations are that physicians are acting in the best interests of all possible future patients. Practically, these studies must be well designed, and all possible pre-study testing must have been done.

SOCIAL SCIENCE

EVIDENCE BASED MEDICINE

BALANCING SCIENTIFIC RESEARCH WITH CLINICAL EXPERIENCE AND PATIENT WISHES

The answers in medicine are never straightforward, no matter how simple the problem may seem. Despite what you might be led to believe, it is neither practical, nor sometimes possible, to solve every problem through deduction, reasoning, and first principles. There are always many variables at play. Juggling uncertainty and balancing risks is one of the key skills of an accomplished doctor.

Where then should a doctor look for guidance when they find their own experience lacking? Should they consult the existing and extensive repertoire of scientific literature? With sometimes many hundreds, if not thousands, of primary research papers written on any given subject, often conflicting with each other, it can be difficult to draw any definitive conclusions. What's more, the patient whose care you are providing, may disagree with your recommendation.

The principle of evidence-based medicine seeks to balance all these considerations when making recommendations for patient care. Largely advocated by Professor Archie Cochrane, a Scottish epidemiologist, the concept of evidence-based medicine has been evolving since the mid-20th century and is now recognised as an important tool in providing effective patient centred care.

Many Cochrane Centres around the world now contribute to a library of so called "Cochrane Reviews" that each seek to appraise a specific clinical question or situation. They achieve this by systematically reviewing all the available data presented in clinical research papers and weighing up their conclusions using a statistical technique called meta-analysis. All this is then balanced with expert and patient opinion to provide clear and concise recommendations to clinicians.

PRINCIPLES OF STATISTICS

PROVIDING THE DATA FOR EVIDENCE BASED MEDICINE

When faced with a problem, best practise is to consult all available data, weigh it up and come to a conclusive answer. This is rarely practical, feasible, or affordable. In such cases a subset of the data (a sample) is studied, and population level conclusions are inferred. If these conclusions are to be true, the sample must be representative of the population.

Testing the relationship between two groups of data is the most common use of statistics. A hypothesis (the 'alternative' hypothesis) is proposed about the relationship between the groups of data (e.g. men are taller than women). Contrasting this hypothesis is another one (the 'null' hypothesis) that states there is no difference between the groups. It is far easier to disprove a fact than provide incontrovertible proof that it is true, hence statistical tests aim to disprove (reject) the null hypothesis and quantify the level of confidence assigned to this rejection.

The level of confidence in the result of a statistical test (e.g. in rejecting a null hypothesis and stating that there is a difference between two groups) is expressed as a p-value. Specifically, the p-value is the probability of getting the observed results when the null hypothesis (that there is no difference) is true. A low p-value indicates it is unlikely that the observed results happened by chance and supports the rejection of the null hypothesis.

In science, we typically say results are statistically significant if the p-value is less than 0.05 (less than 5% chance that these results would be observed if there was no real difference between groups). Whether this has a 'real-life' impact is another question; in medicine this real-life impact if referred to as clinical significance.

> Clinical significance relies on the effect size i.e. the absolute difference between two groups. If there is a small p-value then the results are not likely to be due to change. However, if this result indicates a significant, but very small difference between two groups, it may not be clinically significant as it is too small to be of any practical value. A statistically significant, but not clinically significant difference would be if a treatment reduced a patient's rating of pain from 9.5/10 to 9.4/10 with a p-value of 0.04. At this point, we would question whether it was worth implementing this treatment, especially if it was expensive.

MEASURING DISEASE BURDEN

QUANTIFICATION OF YEARS LOST DUE TO DISEASE

Years lost to disease is a concept used in public health to help understand the impact of a disease. The two main quantification measures are quality-adjusted life years (QALYs) and disability-adjusted life years (DALYs).

The **QALY** was first used in the 1970's, and by the mid 90's was widely accepted as the gold-standard in cost-effectiveness analysis. QALYs are a product of the number of years lived in a given state of health and the utility score attributed to this given state (years of life x utility score). The utility score is a number between 0 (death) and 1 (perfect health), hence one QALY signifies one year lived in perfect health. One way to calculate the utility score is using the EQ-5D questionnaire that measures health status based on five aspects.

The **DALY** was developed in the 1990's and represents loss of healthy life due to disease. It is used as a societal measure to demonstrate health gaps. It is calculated by the sum of years of life lost (YLL), and years of life lost to disability (YLD). YLD measures the burden of living with the condition and includes an adjustment for the severity of the condition (similar to the utility score in QALYs).

Various issues exist around measuring disease burden. The method of adjustment based on the nature of the condition is subject to debate. In DALYs, criticism is levied at the idea that there should be age-weighting with respect to years lived as a young adult counting more than years lived as an older adult. In addition, neither DALYs or QALYs can truly capture the wider effect to the individual or society occur due to health events.

> 10 years lived in a state health with a utility score of 0.7 would generate 7 QALYs. If a treatment increased the utility score over this time to 0.8, then over ten years, an extra QALY has been generated. If one year of treatment cost £5,000, the cost per QALY is £50,000. This is the basis of cost-effectiveness analysis to compare different treatments. Proponents of this method argue it allows more optimisation of societal benefit from limited health resources.

NUMBER NEEDED TO TREAT

A STATISTICAL MEASURE THAT GIVES INFORMATION ABOUT THE EFFECTIVENESS OF MEDICAL TREATMENTS.

The number need to treat (NNT) is defined as the number of patients that must be treated with a new treatment in order for one *extra* person to benefit compared to the standard treatment.

> An illustrative example: imagine a fictional treatment for heart attacks called 'HeartSaver'. Of those that are given HeartSaver when they have a heart attack, 75% survive (25% die). Of those who are given nothing when they have a heart attack, 25% survive (75% die). HeartSaver saved the lives of 50% of people who took it but did nothing to help the 25% who would have survived anyway (without treatment), nor the 25% who died regardless of being given the treatment. Hence, there is a 50% absolute risk reduction and therefore we can express this as having to treat two people in order for the treatment to affect 1 person. Hence the NNT is 2.

The NNT is used in combination with information about a treatments cost to determine what treatments the NHS will provide. An expensive treatment with a very high NNT may not be provided.

A further factor is that the NNT does not account for side effects. A treatment may be very effective and have a low NNT, but if the side effect profile is severe then it may not be used.

There are a number of considerations to be made about the NNT:

- The NNT is a comparative measure, therefore what the comparator is matters. E.g. an incumbent treatment, a placebo, or no treatment at all (as in the example above).
- If the clinical endpoint is severe enough (such as a heart attack), drugs with a high NNT may still be indicated even if they are expensive.
- The benefit a treatment confers does not have to be the preservation of life (as it is in the above example).

SENSITIVITY AND SPECIFICITY

USED TO EVALUATE HOW GOOD A DIAGNOSTIC TEST IS

Sensitivity measures how good a test is at detecting something *if it is present* (i.e. how often a test will have a positive result in a person that has a disease – true positive result). **Specificity** is how often a test will correctly identify the *absence* of something (i.e. how often a test will have a negative result in a person that doesn't have a disease – true negative result).

Both sensitivity and specificity are expressed as a number between 0 and 1, or as a percentage between 0% and 100%. The higher the number, the better the test. The formulas of the above descriptions are:

Sensitivity = Σ True positive test results/Σ Number of sick people

Specificity = Σ True negative test results/Σ Number of healthy people

99.9% sensitivity (remember this refers to true positive results) means that if 1000 people have a disease, the investigation that test for the disease will pick this up in 999 of these people. Consequently, 1 person with the disease will have a false negative result.

Sensitivity and specificity are intrinsic properties of how good a test is, and so are independent of the population the test is applied to. On the next page we will discuss how an *individual clinician* interprets the results of a *specific patient's* test result and show why tests may not be as good as high sensitivity and specificity values may imply.

> The sensitivity and specificity of a test form the basis for how we evaluate machine learning powered diagnostic models. Recently, machine learning has been used to diagnose patients from chest radiographs (chest X-rays). The sensitivity and specificity of the machine learning models is calculated by comparing the diagnosis with the gold-standard confirmed diagnoses by biopsies, more detailed scans, consensus of panels of radiologists etc. Because such gold-standard diagnoses can be time consuming or expensive, a machine learning model that is not perfect could be tolerated if it has reasonable sensitivity and specificity.

POSITIVE AND NEGATIVE PREDICTIVE VALUES

INDIVIDUAL CLINICIANS USING DIAGNOSTIC TESTS

This page will use HIV testing to illustrate the difference between the sensitivity of a test and its positive predictive value (PPV). An equivalent idea applies to specificity and negative predictive value (NPV).

In clinical practise, when interpreting a positive test result (e.g. positive HIV test), the crucial question is: "How likely is it that this patient actually has this disease?". If a HIV test has 99.9% sensitivity and 95% specificity (a good test), given the previous page, one may assume a clinician could be 99.9% sure such a patient has HIV. Unfortunately, this is wrong. The PPV (and NPV) are needed to assess the value of a specific test result.

The PPV and NPV represent the *proportion* of positive and negative results that are true positive and negative results, respectively. The PPV formula is:

PPV = Σ true positive results/ Σ positive results

Σ positive results = number of true positives + number of false positives

Crucially, when the prevalence of a disease is low, the number of false positive results is high *relative* to the number of true positives. The false positive rate is 1 − sensitivity (an intrinsic property of the test), whereas the number of true positives depends on sensitivity *and* the prevalence of the disease in the population.

Assume 1 in 100 people in a population have HIV. As sensitivity is above 99%, this test should easily correctly identify all 10 people per 1000 that have HIV. However, the test would also be expected to erroneously identify 50 people per 1000 tested as having HIV when they do not (as specificity is 'only' 95%). In this case, 17% of those with a positive test result have HIV.

It is more dramatic if we now assume 1 in 1000 people have HIV. We would expect the test to identify this person as the sensitivity is 99.9%. However, the test would still be expected to identify 50 people per 1000 tested as having HIV when they do not (specificity is 'only' 99%). In this case, only 2% of those with a positive test result have HIV. Clearly when the prevalence of a disease is low, isolated test results cannot instil confidence, and need further investigation.

SURVIVAL ANALYSIS

TIME TO EVENT ANALYSIS

Survival analysis does not deal exclusively in the analysis of death; the event in question can be survival free of a disease or other specific events. Such a specific event is referred to as an end-point in medical research studies. The analysis is to look at how many end-points have happened in a given time period in two or more different groups of people.

Issues surround survival analysis of clinical trials. These relate to censored data. This is when only partial information is known about an outcome. In survival analysis this is known as Right censoring, and occurs because:

- Patients are 'lost' within the follow-up time, either because researchers can no longer contact them, or because subjects (often patients) ask to leave a trial before they experience an event that may or may not (hence the partial information) have subsequently occurred.
- Patients have not experienced an event when they are last seen for follow-up but are alive and may have gone on to have this had observation continued.

The tool most commonly used in survival analysis is the Kaplan-Meier estimator as it deals well with Right censoring. This used to produce Kaplan-Meier survival curves (shown right). The creating of the estimator (and thus the curves) requires information on each subject about whether either an event or censoring occurred, and the time at which this happened, often given in days post start time. Statistical tests can be applied to determine if the difference between two curves (and thus survival of two groups) is statistically significant.

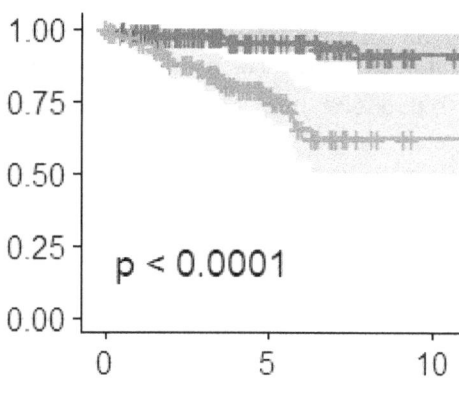

The difference in survival after taking drug A vs drug B is a common use for survival curves. A statistically significant difference between the two generated curves means one drug is *statistically* superior to the other, and the difference observed can be concluded to be real.

HEALTH INEQUALITIES

IMPORTANT IN SOCIETAL DETERMINANTS OF HEALTH

One of the founding principles of the NHS was that it should be equitable, meaning fair and impartial. The NHS has remained largely fair in its treatment of individuals, however there are some wider inequalities in service and in health that are present when looking at a population level.

The most extreme effect of these health inequalities is that there are large differences in life expectancy within the UK; up to 20 years difference between those in the least and most deprived areas. Inequalities also exist in healthy life expectancy, wellbeing and morbidity.

> One often cited example of health inequality is the city of Glasgow. Male life expectancy falls markedly for every station on the trainline in Glasgow that travels from the affluent west side to the less affluent east side, and the male life expectancy in some areas was as low as 55 years. The 'Glasgow effect' is a term used to indicate that this life expectancy and poor health is worse than those in similarly deprived areas of other UK cities.

The 'Marmot indicators' are a range of measures that are used to assess and monitor the level of health inequality in the NHS. These indicators are largely aligned with the six policy recommendations put forward in the 2010 report *'Fair Society Healthy Lives'*. Chief among these recommendations is that every child should be given the best start in life, maximise their capabilities and have control over their lives. This is in line with the theory of salutogenesis, an approach that focuses on factors promoting health and wellbeing, rather than factors directly causing disease (e.g. smoking)

Looking more generally, the fundamental causes of health inequalities include global economic forces, political priorities and resulting decisions, marginalisation, discrimination, and unequal distribution of income and wealth. The latter is the focus of the book *'The Spirit Level'* by Wilkinson and Pickett. The book argues that for a wide range of health and social problem, including physical and mental health, outcomes are significantly worse in more unequal countries, regardless of the overall wealth of the country.

FALLS IN THE ELDERLY

A VERY COMMON CAUSE OF MORBIDITY AND MORTALITY

Falls are common occurrences in the elderly and have profound impact on the individual, their family, and on the health service.

Any writing on falls in the elderly must consider the obvious traumatic consequences that occur. Head injuries and broken bones, especially fractures of the neck of the femur, are commonplace. The latter is potentiated by low bone density in the elderly; osteoporosis is common, especially among women.

> The mortality rate within one year of a fractured neck of femur is around 30%. This figure is likely a factor of the older demographic these fractures commonly happen in, the operation that is often required, and the prolonged stay in hospital that their treatment necessitates. Irrespective, it encapsulates the harm that a fall can cause to an elderly person.

However, the consequences of falls go beyond trauma. Even without injury, falls can lead to a loss of confidence in one's ability to mobilise independently, and a fear of falling again. This can lead to a downward spiral of declining physical health, psychological health, and social activity. Loss of any one of these further potentiates loss of the others, largely through the consequences of inactivity. It is therefore not surprising that some view the start of old age as the time of the first age related fall.

There are things that cause that older people fall. Impaired balance, reduced strength, poor eyesight and polypharmacy are common and significant contributing factors. Polypharmacy is when a person is taking several drugs (the exact number differs in different definitions) at the same time. It is associated with falls as many drugs can be mild sedatives, hypnotics, or can cause hypotension, all of which can increase the risk of falls.

For the health service, falls present a huge challenge. They are the cause of many admissions and cost an enormous amount of money. Measures to prevent them are crucial. Exercise that starts in middle age and continues into older age is a proven way to prevent falls in the elderly.

DRUGS ON PATENT

A MATTER OF COST

The drug research and development pipeline is long, costly, and often unsuccessful. For this reason, companies will file for a patent soon after discovery of a molecule with a novel mechanism of action. This is seen as important as it provides financial incentive for innovation. After a patent is granted, companies have exclusive rights to supply the molecule as a drug for 20 years. The drug is known as 'proprietary' and is sold under a brand name. After the patent expires, competitors can enter the market with generic drugs that are sold at lower prices and therefore offer significant benefits to societal supply.

A generic drug is a drug that contains the chemical compound (active pharmaceutical ingredient) that was originally protected by patent. Other aspects of the generic drug may differ (the inactive ingredients) and the price is typically much lower. This means it can be prescribed more widely. Atorvastatin is one of the most commonly used drugs in the world. It is a statin originally developed by Pfizer and used in cardiovascular preventative medicine. Until 2012, it was under patent in the UK and sold under the brand name Lipitor. After the loss of patent, the price of the drug reduced by as much as 85%.

Given the loss of profit-making ability once a proprietary drug comes 'off-patent' (known as the patent cliff) there are significant efforts made to extend patents. There are a number of technical, legal, and business orientated ways that this can happen, and the process is known 'evergreening'.

> Insulin is a peptide hormone produced by the pancreas that helps lower blood sugar levels. In type 1 diabetes, the cells that produce insulin are destroyed. In 1921, Banting and Best isolated insulin from a dog's pancreas at Toronto university. The university held the patent, licensed drug companies to manufacture it and gave them the rights to themselves patent any improvements. To this day, Insulin remains a very expensive medication, especially in America. This is because incremental innovation and subsequent patenting has been a form of 'evergreening' that means that there is still no generic insulin in America.

TECHNOLOGY IN HEALTHCARE

APPLYING TECHNOLOGICAL INNOVATION TO PATIENT CARE

Moore's Law states that every two years the average transistor size halves, meaning the transistor density on a single microchip doubles. This reflects the fact that roughly every other year the computational power of silicon semiconductors doubles, and existing processors halve in size, thereby dramatically reducing their cost. Moore's Law and the exponential growth it describes has underpinned the rapid development of computer science in recent decades. To put this into perspective a fairly average modern smart phone contains many thousand times more processing power than the computers on board the Apollo 11 mission to the moon!

Despite this rapid evolution of technology, it can be a slow process to see it transition to the application of healthcare. This is a common theme in healthcare where there is often resistance to novel techniques and technologies in favour of tried and tested methods. Whilst it is true that new developments may present unknown risks to patients (for example Thalidomide), it may also convey significant benefits (for example laparoscopic surgery). Therefore, a key part of modern medicine is providing a platform for the safe trialling of novel technology, techniques and drugs.

An example of a rapidly evolving concept in healthcare is the application of artificial intelligence (AI). A large part of research in medicine is identifying patterns and trends, often empirically, to then fit to a biological model. In many cases these patterns can be too complex for the human mind to spot. AI is one solution to this problem. By providing a computer with a sufficiently large dataset it can spot patterns for itself, generating infinitely complex algorithms to fit the data presented to it. These algorithms can then be applied to novel situations to solve problems. For example, after being shown 10,000 pictures of cats, and 10,000 pictures of dogs, the Google "Deep Mind" AI could distinguish between a cat and a dog 70% of the time.

There are perhaps some obvious applications of this technique in radiology. Automating the process of analysing complex medical imaging could save time, remove human error, and cut costs. The use of AI in reading mammograms to identify breast cancers and identifying lung cancers from chest x-rays, for example, has already made headlines. However, there are some lesser appreciated applications of AI which are rapidly developing. Most notably in the creation of so called "smart prosthetics". By teaching a robotic prosthesis to identify normal gait, researchers have been able to build a prosthetic leg that could even identify an imminent fall and correct a stumbling patient.

STRUCTURE OF THE HEALTH SERVICE

THE FORMATION OF THE NHS

THE UNIVERSAL HEALTHCARE SYSTEM

On July 5th, 1948, Aneurin (Nye) Bevan, the then Labour health minister, launched the NHS at Park Hospital in Manchester (now Trafford General Hospital). This marked a shift from healthcare that was for those who could afford it to a service that was accessible to all, irrespective of background. The service was to be provided free at the point of use, financed by central taxation, and everyone (even those visiting the country) would be eligible for care.

Following the start of the Second World War, a free Emergency Hospital Service had been created. As this was operating, the White Paper titled "A National Health Service" was published in 1944 by the Conservative government. In the 1945 General Election that was won by Labour, both Conservative and Labour parties committed to free access to health care service, and in 1946 The National Health Service Act was published. This set out the terms that health care would be provided free of charge, except in specific circumstances explicitly outlined in the Act.

In 1948, following two years of debate with doctors who worried about loss of independence and earning powers, Nye Bevan launched the NHS and described it as "the biggest single experiment in social services that the world has ever seen". The NHS has undergone numerous reforms since inception, but its ongoing survival has been a remarkable success.

> "It will provide you with all medical, dental and nursing care. Everyone — rich or poor, man, woman or child — can use it or any part of it. There are no charges, except for a few special items. There are no insurance qualifications. But it is not a "charity". You are all paying for it, mainly as tax-payers, and it will relieve your money worries in time of illness."
> Central Office of Information, for the Ministry of Health.

PRIMARY, SECONDARY AND TERTIARY CARE

A BASIC BUT ESSENTIAL FRAMEWORK OF THE NHS

Primary care encompasses the services that a person usually first sees when they are unwell. This is normally a GP or practise nurse but could be a number of other professionals who are normally based in the community. NHS direct, walk-in centres, dentists and opticians also fall under the banner of primary care. By and large, primary care practitioners are generalists and will refer on to specialist care if needed.

Secondary care is largely based in hospitals and deals with issues that cannot be resolved in primary care. A referral from primary care is required to be treated in secondary care, and it is often delivered via hospital clinic appointments. Treatment is done by consultant specialising in one area of medicine and involves medication, surgery, or occasionally conservative treatment. These hospitals are often district general hospitals based in towns or small cities.

Accident and Emergency departments lie on the boundary of primary and secondary care.

Tertiary care is healthcare provided in specialist national or regional centres. Referrals may come straight from primary care but are often received via secondary care from centres not able to deal with a complex case. Tertiary care centres will have all available treatments and methods of investigations and are often based in large cities which act as regional hubs.

> Adam is a 12 year old boy who notices a painful area on his knee but assumes it is from playing football. Two weeks later there is slight raising of the area, so his parents take him to see their GP. The GP refers them onto the local hospital for an X-ray. The doctors there then refer the family onto the large hospital in the local city for further imaging, a biopsy and immunohistochemical analysis which confirms a diagnosis of Ewing's sarcoma. Adam stays attached to the tertiary site for the duration of his chemotherapy treatment and surgical resection.

FUNDING THE NHS

FREE AT THE POINT OF CARE, PAID FOR IN TAXATION

One defining feature of the NHS is that it is free at the point of care.

The NHS budget is funded primarily by general taxation and national insurance contributions deducted from those earning over a set amount. This changes annually and is subject to regular review. Funding from taxation and national insurance accounts for approximately 99% of the NHS budget. The remainder is provided by charges made to patients for things like prescriptions (but not in Wales), parking charges, and appointments with the dentists and opticians.

Quite how much each of these revenues will accrue is somewhat unknown and thus every year the government conducts a spending review process to predict the total income. The government works on a budget of approximately £2,200 per person and so for example the expected NHS spending in 2020 was predicted to be £123 billion. Generally, if there is a predicted shortfall the difference is made up by redirecting general taxation income previously assigned to other services.

The budget is broken down into investing in capital, and day to day expenditure. Investing in capital accounts for 10% of the budget and includes spending on new hospitals, public health initiatives, and training. Day to day running of the NHS such as staff pay, equipment, and medicines takes the remaining money.

Funding is allocated to Clinical Commissioning Groups (CCG's) based on a "weighted capitation" resources formula which essentially aims to direct resources to where they are needed most.

Once the money has been awarded to the CCG's it is their responsibility to construct their own budget and allocate funds. Over 50% of this is normally awarded to acute health services such as hospitals.

DISTRIBUTION OF NHS FUNDS

FLOW OF MONEY IN THE NHS

The structure of the NHS and flow of money between parts of it was overhauled in the Health and Social Care Act 2012 and is now quite convoluted.

The department for health is a governmental department that is responsible for policy to improve the quality of care delivered. The department has a number of public bodies that it oversees including the National Institute for Health and Care Excellence (NICE), Health Education England, NHS Digital, the Care Quality Commission, and NHS England.

NHS England (NHS commissioning board) overseas the budget and commissioning (buying of services) of the NHS. NHS England commissions specialised services accounting for about 15% of the NHS budget, allocates about 65% of the NHS budget to clinical commissioning groups (CCGs), and holds the employment contracts for GPs, dentists, opticians and pharmacists.

A clinical commissioning group is made up of local GPS, secondary care consultants, and lay members. Each group is in charge of commissioning most primary and secondary care services in that region (excluding the specialist services that NHS England commissions). CCGs are required to assess local needs and decide on what is important, and then set strategies to meet this need.

The providers of healthcare are the primary, secondary and tertiary services. Most secondary and tertiary care is provided by NHS foundation trusts, but also by private companies, voluntary services, and other non-NHS providers.

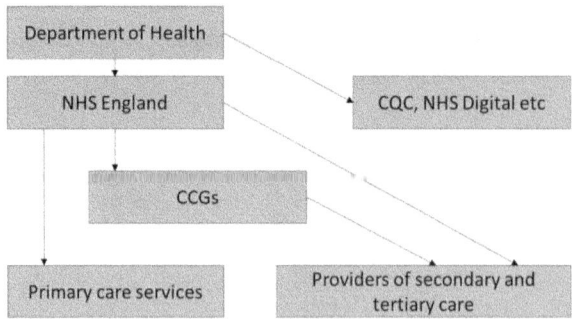

ALLIED HEALTH PROFESSIONALS

HEALTH PROFESSIONALS DISTINCT FROM DOCTORS AND NURSES

The medical team is large and there are many different roles within it. Allied Health Professionals (AHPs) are professionally autonomous practitioners who use their expertise to diagnose, treat and prevent disease in patients.

In the NHS there are 14 recognised AHP roles; art therapists; dieticians; drama therapists; music therapists; occupational therapists; operating department practitioners; orthoptists; osteopaths; paramedics; physiotherapists; podiatrists; prosthetists and orthotists; radiographers; speech and language therapists.

These are protected professional titles and anyone using one must be registered with the relevant professional body. Of the 14 AHP roles, 13 are regulated by the Health and Care Professions Council (HCPC) with Osteopaths regulated by the General Osteopathic Council (GOC).

Doctors work alongside AHPs and utilise their expertise. In the NHS Long Term Plan, AHPs will take an increasing role in improving health and social care across hospitals and communities, acting as a first-point-of-contact that will enable faster diagnostics and earlier intervention.

> Dieticians translate the science of nutrition into patient care. They work with patients with chronic health problems that mean their nutrition can be compromised, or those who have been acutely unwell. Specific examples include gastroenterology patients, intensive care patients, HIV patients, cancer patients, and patients with eating disorders. In addition, dieticians are crucial for public health initiates centred around diet and obesity.

ASYLUM SEEKERS ENTITLEMENT TO NHS SERVICES

PEOPLE SEEKING ASYLUM CAN FACE BARRIERS TO ACCESS

An asylum seeker is a person seeking protection from persecution abroad. They may leave their country due to fear of serious harm, torture, inhumane treatment, or punishment. Such people enter another country as an immigrant, and apply for asylum status, which if granted will mean they are considered a refugee, at which point they are eligible for mainstream benefits and have the right to work.

The rules are clear. Anyone can access primary care for free, and a lack of ID or proof of address should not prevent registration at a GP practice. Lack of address or ID can indicate a person is in a vulnerable situation, and therefore it is crucial that they can access the care they need.

Secondary care is more complex and treated differently to primary care. Unless a person is considered 'ordinarily resident' (a legal concept affecting entitlement to the NHS), they must pay for secondary care up-front. There are exceptions to this monetary requirement based on the status of the patient (e.g. asylum seekers, refugees, those on a work/student visa) and on the type of medical care. Urgent care (as defined by a clinician) and maternity treatment must never be withheld although can be charged later, and certain services remain free to all (e.g. A&E, treatment for infectious diseases such as TB and sexually transmitted infections, and palliative care).

The summary for asylum seekers and refugees is that they are entitled to all NHS services that are free of charge to UK residents.

> Doctors of the World are a charity that performs healthcare work around the world. Their UK-based work focusses on clinics and advocacy programmes in London to support healthcare for people on the margins of society, including destitute migrants, sex workers, and those with no fixed abode. The patients they treat are often fully entitled to mainstream healthcare, but do not engage with it due to fear, having to pay, or being turned away incorrectly by frontline health staff.

THE MEDICAL CAREER PATHWAY

A VARIED PATH

Climbing through the ranks in medicine as a doctor is very much a marathon and not a sprint, potentially requiring decades of postgraduate training and exams. The options available to medical graduates are large, but for a doctor the basic career structure remains the same.

Medical school marks the start of the process. This is either an undergraduate course lasting five or six years, or a post graduate course typically lasting four years. Many undergraduate courses now offer the opportunity to intercalate, meaning that you may take a year out from medicine in order to study for another degree that compliments or contrasts what you have already learnt.

After graduating from medical school, provisional registration with the General Medical Council (GMC) is granted before entering onto one of the many types of foundation programme. It is at this point that you become a "resident doctor", and this, rather strangely, remains the overarching title until a consultant post is achieved. Foundation programmes last two years (FY1 and FY2) and are analogous to an apprenticeship with a pro rata salary and on the job experience. Normally full GMC registration is awarded at the end of FY1.

After completion of foundation training, a doctor commences specialty training. This can be broken in two, composed of a "core" specialty training programme, followed by re-application to a "higher" specialty training programme. Alternatively, specialty training programmes can be described as "run through", which do not require any re-application and instead, once you're accepted onto a programme, your progression is automatic if you meet the required competencies along the way. For most specialties this takes between five and seven years, however for general practice it only takes three.

Once specialty training is complete a senior clinical position can be obtained as a consultant. The fastest this can be achieved is training to be a general practitioner (GP). This can take ten years at a minimum (5 in medical school, 2 foundation and 3 specialty GP training), meaning full qualification by a minimum age of 28.

Many doctors will spend time on this pathway earning extra degrees, taking time out for research, maternity leave, or undertaking fellowships to learn advanced skills, meaning there is huge variation in the specific experience people collect throughout training.

APPLYING TO MEDICINE (UK)

A BASIC OVERVIEW OF THE PROCESS

The submission, or consideration, of an application to medical school is likely why you are reading this book. Whether you are a school leaver or graduate dictates the details of the universities you can apply to, and the requirements needed. We will try to outline generalisable themes rather than specifics, and as such this should be useful to both cohorts.

In general, your application to a medical school is made with intention of securing an interview, after which point the slate is normally 'wiped clean' and offers are given out based on merit at the interview. The application consists of your academic results, scores in the various admission tests, and finally your personal statement.

Preparation is key to your success. It is crucial to research the courses sufficiently in order that you can apply your strengths to applications. This means that you stand a higher chance of getting an interview, and therefore an offer, if you research *exactly* what each university prioritise when calling candidates for interview, and then apply to universities that match with what you have done well in.

Preparation for the admissions tests is strongly encouraged. There is no absolute need to have tuition for this, but focussed and diligent individual preparation is essential.

Quantity of work experience is something that can cause concern among applicants. It is accepted that work experience can be hard to get, in particular in hospitals where organisation is often through personal networks. This is to the detriment of those from less affluent backgrounds.

It is the opinion of the authors that quality of engagement with the experience and subsequent reflection upon it trumps quantity of experience. Furthermore, we believe an applicant can demonstrate better commitment with a period of work in a nursing home than any number of weeks shadowing hospital consultants.

TWO-WEEK WAIT PATHWAY

FOR THE DETECTION OF CANCER

The NHS constitution sets out the rights for patients with suspected cancer to be seen by a cancer specialist within a maximum of two weeks from GP referral for urgent referrals where cancer is suspected. The process by which this happens is known as The Two Week Wait Referral Service (2WW), and involves referring from primary care to secondary care.

More than 300,000 new cancers across over 200 different cancer types are diagnosed in the UK each year. Each cancer type will present differently but there are often overlapping features, especially among those cancers which affect a particular site. The symptoms that are associated with cancer are classically called "red flag symptoms". Some non-specific red flag symptoms are unexplained weight loss, abnormal bleeding, fatigue, unexplained lumps, loss of appetite. Other red-flag symptoms are specific to the affected tissue.

Once a GP makes the decision to refer on the 2WW pathway, they should endeavour to undertake all investigations their practise can reasonably do. For instance, if a referral is made for suspected prostate cancer (visible blood in urine, issues with urinating, erectile dysfunction) the GP should request a prostate-specific antigen blood test, take the blood from the patient, and send it for analysis such that the result will be ready by the time the specialist appointment happens. This streamlines the process and gives the cancer specialist (a urologist in this case) the maximum amount of information when they meet the patient. Many of the patients referred on the 2WW pathway do not have cancer, but if they do they will undergo further specialist care.

> The colorectal cancer referral pathway states to refer patients for an appointment within 2 weeks if they are aged 40 and over with unexplained weight loss and abdominal pain *or* they are aged 50 and over with unexplained rectal bleeding *or* they are aged 60 and over with iron deficiency anaemia/ changes in their bowel habit *or* if at any age a test shows occult blood in the faeces.

HISTORY OF MEDICINE

BEAUMONT & ST MARTIN

ETHICAL STANDARDS HAVE EVOLVED

The evolution of medicine and our understanding of physiology has at times been driven by practice that by modern standard is considered unethical. This is exemplified no better than in the case of Beaumont and St Martin.

Whilst practicing as a surgeon, William Beaumont (1785 – 1853) saved the life of Alexis St Martin after he sustained a gunshot wound to the abdomen. Over the subsequent days the wound healed as a permanent hole connecting St Martin's stomach with the outside world. This type of wound is known as a gastrocutaneous fistula. This presented Beaumont with a window into the inner workings of St Martin's bowels at a time when there was no scientific understanding of digestion.

Beaumont recognised this and seized his chance by persuading the oblivious and illiterate St Martin to sign a contract binding him as Beaumont's servant. Whilst the majority of his chores where those mundane and expected of servants, he was also obliged to participate in Beaumont's experiments. Many of which involved stuffing food tied to a string through St Martin's wound and directly into his stomach. By later pulling the string out Beaumont was literally able to watch digestion happening.

> Today, Beaumont's work has resurfaced as some of the first evidence of a psychophysiological gut response. Specifically, Beaumont noted the impact of emotional arousal on rate of digestion and gut motility. When St Martin was stressed, or agitated digestion was much slower.
>
> This concept of a gut-brain axis is very topical at the moment since a number of researchers have shown that this communication can occur in reverse. With the food we eat and the bacteria in our gut having the power to change our mood!

Over the many experiments Beaumont performed on St Martin, he made inroads into understanding the physiology of digestion. Whilst this arguably paved the way for the current specialty of gastroenterology, it came at much discomfort for St Martin. Needless to say, this would not be granted ethical approval today!

EDWARD JENNER

THE FATHER OF IMMUNOLOGY

Smallpox was an infectious disease, transmitted by one of two viral variants, which devastated mankind for centuries. In the 18th century smallpox was rife, killing over 400,000 people annually across Europe. Those infected were named "speckled monsters" and anywhere up to 60% of adults and 98% of infants would die. Of those who survived, a third would go blind.

Despite the staggering death toll, by the early 1700s the process of "variolation" or inoculation was gaining traction. It was hoped that by injecting pus from a smallpox blister into a pocket under the skin a localised infection would convey immunity. However, more often than not, this would lead to disseminated small pox infection with the associated mortality, although if patients survived, they were immune.

Edward Jenner, born 17th May 1749, a doctor living and working in Gloucestershire, had heard for many years how dairymaids were protected from smallpox if they had suffered cowpox – a rarely fatal disease. Jenner postulated that cowpox could be utilised in the variolation method of inoculation to convey protection against smallpox.

In May 1796 Jenner tested his hypothesis by extracting fluid from a dairymaid's cowpox blisters before injecting it into 8-year-old James Phipps' arm. Subsequently James developed a fever, but when Jenner inoculated the boy again a month later, this time with pus from a fresh smallpox blister, no disease developed. James was immune.

Jenner did not know the biology behind the process, but termed the treatment a vaccine, after the Latin for cow 'vacca'. Jenner's discovery of vaccination paved the way for a new field of medicine that has subsequently saved millions of lives. As for smallpox; the last case of naturally occurring smallpox was diagnosed in October 1977 and in 1980 the World Health Organisation announced its total eradication.

ROBERT LISTON

A PIONEER OF ANAESTHESIA

Robert Liston born 1794, was a surgeon described as "the fastest knife in the West-End". In a time before anaesthesia, when speed of operation was regarded as the key factor in patient recovery, he was famed for having amputated a leg in 28 seconds, and on another occasion removed a 10kg scrotal tumour in under 4 minutes. The later liberated the patient from the wheelbarrow that was used to aid transportation.

However, his haste did not come without consequence. Arguably Liston's most famous case was the amputation of a gangrenous leg in which he inadvertently slashed through his assistant's fingers, the sight of which caused an observer to die of a heart attack. Over the subsequent days both Liston's patient and assistant developed sepsis and died. To this day, Liston remains the only surgeon in history to have conducted an operation with a 300% mortality rate!

Despite this reputation, on the 21st of December 1846, Robert Liston became the first surgeon in Europe to conduct an operation under modern anaesthesia. Following on from the success of the dentist, William Morton in Boston, Liston adopted the use of a substance called ether to anaesthetise a patient for leg amputation.

Whilst this heralded a new era in surgery, it actually increased patient mortality. Without the screams of their patients, surgeons grew ever more adventurous in a time where germ theory was not known. The field of surgery still had a lot more to learn.

IGNAZ SEMMELWEIS

"SAVIOUR OF MOTHERS"

Ignaz Semmelweis was a Hungarian doctor working in the Vienna General Hospital during the mid 1800s. He his famed for his early work on the concept of hand hygiene stemming from his observations of maternal deaths due to puerperal fever (otherwise known as "childbed fever").

At the time, expectant mothers in Vienna would be admitted to one of two clinics. The first had a mortality rate of over 10% whereas in the second only 4% of mothers were dying of puerperal fever. Semmelweis noted this to be strange given the environment and procedures carried out in each clinic were identical. Moreover, this the public were aware of this, and Semmelweis would frequently find mothers requesting to be admitted to the second clinic.

The only discernible difference between the two clinics was that the first was attended by medical students, and the second by student midwives. Semmelweis' observed that the medical students conducted autopsies immediately prior to attending maternity clinics, whereas the student midwives had no exposure to cadaveric material. Hence Semmelweis proposed that the medical students were carrying "cadaveric particles" on their hands which were transferred to the expectant mothers.

Semmelweis began to advocate the washing of hands in chlorinated lime solution before proceeding from the autopsy lab to the maternity clinic. In 1847, he published his first results claiming to have reduced the mortality to below 1%. Unfortunately, this was a time when germ theory did not exist and Semmelweis could not explain the science underpinning his work.

Many of his medical colleagues ridiculed him and he was later admitted to an asylum where he died of sepsis following a savage beating. It was only after the work of Louis Pasteur that Semmelweis' genius was recognised and implemented in modern clinical practice.

JOHN SNOW

ONE OF THE FATHERS OF EPIDEMIOLOGY

The year is 1854 and an outbreak of cholera is rife in Soho, London. At the time the accepted theory of disease was miasma; the germ theory of disease was only slowly gaining traction and had not formally been proposed by Pasteur. The miasma theory held that diseases (such as cholera) were caused by a form of 'bad air' that originated from rotting organic matter.

John Snow was a physician sceptical of the miasma theory. He believed sewage dumped near wells and water supplies could cause cholera outbreaks. Snow was working in Soho in 1854 and began investigating the cholera outbreak. He saw that fatalities were centred around Broad Street and set about painstakingly enquiring about whether those that were infected had drunk water from the water pump on Broad Street. He drew a now famous map, depicting the clusters of cholera cases in the Soho outbreak. Snow collected enough evidence to persuade the authorities to remove the handle from the pump, and shortly after this the outbreak came to an end. Whilst the epidemic was in decline before the handle was removed, it was the logical analysis and pragmatic response that means this event is seminal in the history of public health.

Epidemiology is the study of the distribution of disease. Today it relies heavily on statistics to analyse population level amounts of data and goes hand in hand with public health. It is therefore fitting that Snow, with his map (a form of data analysis), and his influence on the removal of the handle, be seen as one of the fathers of modern epidemiology.

> Google Flu Trends was a modern day version of Snow's map. Google tracks all searches made by its users. In the 2009 flu pandemic (see page __) Google tracked searches for flu associated symptoms and the location this search was made from. Some estimates predicted Google Flu could predict outbreaks ten days before the American CDC (Centre for Disease Control and Prevention).

ASEPTIC TECHNIQUE

APPLYING GERM THEORY TO SURGICAL PRACTICE

During the mid-19th century, following the discovery of anaesthesia, going under the surgeon's knife was more dangerous than ever. No longer deterred by the struggles and screams of their patients, surgeons became bolder and more adventurous. Often cramming their operating lists with so many patients they lacked the time to wash their hands or instruments between cases. In a time when little was known about the transmission of disease, the incidence of post operative infections soared with lethal consequences.

Hope for patients came in 1862 through the work of Joseph Lister and his application of the work of the French microbiologist, Louis Pasteur. Pasteur had already suggested the role of bacteria in causing disease and had even successfully prolonged the life of milk and wine through his own sterilisation technique – pasteurisation. Lister surmised that if bacterial contamination was the cause for disease, then the suppuration seen in surgical wounds could be prevented with an analogous sterilisation procedure. The trick would be finding a method that was lethal to bacteria but safe for the patient.

Drawing on his observations from the agricultural industry Lister settled on the organic aromatic chemical phenol, or carbolic acid. The opportunity to test his theory arose in August 1865, when an 11-year-old boy presented with an open fracture after his leg was run over by a horse and cart. In Lister's time this was a catastrophic injury, with the certainty of infection, necessitating immediate amputation of the whole leg if life was to be preserved.

Lister stayed his knife and instead applied a lint cloth soaked in carbolic acid solution to the wound. At 4 days Lister was amazed to see the total absence of infection. He renewed the carbolic acid solution at regular intervals until at 6 weeks not only was the wound free of infection, but the fracture had fully healed. The implications of Lister's discovery were ground-breaking. He immediately ordered all surgeons working under his supervision to wash both their hands and instruments with carbolic acid solution between cases, as well donning clean gloves and spraying carbolic acid vapour over the operative field. Rates of post-operative infection plummeted.

The practice of asepsis has come a long way since the 1860s, with modern operating theatres utilising techniques such as autoclave to sterilise surgical instruments and laminar airflows to carry pathogens away from the operating table. But irrefutably, it is Lister's discovery that has helped to save the lives of thousands of patients. It is not surprising that he is granted the title: the father of modern surgery.

MARIE CURIE

EARLY APPLICATIONS OF RADIOACTIVITY IN MEDICINE

Marie Curie, born Marya Sklodowska in Warsaw in 1867, remains the only person in history to have received two Nobel prizes in two separate scientific categories for her work on radioactivity. At the age of 24 she enrolled at the Sorbonne University in Paris since her own country did not permit the entrance of female students to university. Her career that followed would not just revolutionise the scientific community but also the field of medicine.

Following on from Henri Becquerel's discovery of radioactivity in uranium, Curie quickly discovered a second element some 400 times more radioactive. She named it after her home country, polonium. In later years, Curie identified radium, which was yet more radioactive. Of note, it was through her work on radium that she became one of the first to suggest that atoms were, in fact, not indivisible or inert.

Curie strongly believed that scientific research was, in the economic sense, a public service and sought practical and medical applications for her research. Along with her husband, the Curie's discovered that the radiation from radium killed diseased human cells faster than healthy ones. From this observation the Curie's advocated the use of radiation in the treatment of tumours and developed a rudimentary form of radiotherapy. In later years, following William Roentgen's discovery of x-rays, Curie applied radium to power the world's first medical x-ray machine.

During these early years of studying radioactivity, little was known about the health risks of radiation. Curie was plagued throughout her career by radiation sickness and the aplastic anaemia which killed her in 1934 was undoubtedly caused by a career of unshielded radiation exposure.

> Curie's remains, interred at the Panthèon in Paris, along with all her books, papers, and equipment remain radioactive to this day. All deemed too dangerous to handle, they are kept in lead lined boxes.

THE DISCOVERY OF DNA

BASIC KNOWLEDGE OF DNA STRUCTURE

In popular culture, the story of the discovery of DNA is often near synonymous with the names James Watson and Francis Crick. However, this remarkable story is one that begun almost a century before 1953, the year they reached their famous conclusion that the shape of the DNA molecule is a double helix.

In 1869, Friedrich Miescher discovered a new substance with high phosphate levels (what we know as the sugar-phosphate backbone) inside the nuclei of human cells. He named this molecule 'nuclein'. This term subsequently evolved to 'nucleic acid', and then 'deoxyribonucleic acid (DNA)'.

Various people then began investigating this so called nuclein. In 1919, Phoebus Levene proposed that nuclein was formed of nucleotides, each of which was made of a phosphate group, a sugar group, and one of 4 'bases' (now known as adenine, thymine, guanine, and cytosine). Erwin Chargaff then showed that in a given DNA molecule, the amount of thymine and adenine is equal, and the amount of guanine and cytosine is equal. This is the basis for 'Chargaff's rule', that a molecule of double-stranded DNA has percentage base pair equality.

In the early 1950's, Rosalind Franklin and Maurice Wilkins used x-ray crystallography to produce two high-resolution photos of DNA fibres. Franklin used this to deduce that the phosphates were likely on the outside of a helical-like structure.

Watson and Crick were shown this work, which together with Chargaff's rule allowed them to use cardboard cut-outs to create the famous double helix shape that DNA takes. In 1953, Franklin and Wilkins published their x-ray data in the same Nature issue that Watson and Crick published the structure of DNA. Franklin died in 1958, and so due to a rule barring posthumous presentation, the Nobel Prize in Physiology or Medicine was awarded to Watson, Crick and Wilkins in 1962.

> Linus Pauling is the only person to have ever received two unshared Nobel Prizes (Chemistry in 1954 and Peace in 1962). He proposed the triple helix structure of DNA with the bases on the outside and phosphate on the inside. It was the X-ray crystallography images that allowed Watson and Crick to ultimately pursue the structure that proved correct.

THALIDOMIDE

A BIRTH DEFECT CRISIS

In 1956, Thalidomide emerged as a sedative drug, intended primarily for the treatment of morning sickness in pregnant mothers. What followed is a tragic five-year narrative before a connection was made between prenatal Thalidomide use and profound new-born birth defects affecting somewhere between 10 and 20 thousand babies.

Thalidomide is a stereoisomer that is manufactured as a racemic mixture. Whilst the (R)-enantiomer indeed conveys the intended sedative effects, the (S)-enantiomer is teratogenic, disrupting normal foetal development. Under the biological conditions of the human body the isomers freely convert so separating them is futile.

(R)-Enantiomer   *(S)*-Enantiomer

Thalidomide causes many foetal developmental abnormalities ranging from brain damage to stunted limbs, all dependant on when in pregnancy the foetus is exposed. Only half of Thalidomide babies survived infancy with fewer than 3,000 alive today.

The Thalidomide scandal prompted a global review of pharmaceutical licensing policies with the 1968 Medicines Act introduced in the UK; frameworks which still guide and influence current medical practice.

> Thalidomide is still used in clinical practice today for the treatment of myeloma and leprosy, although its use in women of childbearing age is understandably tightly regulated.

PIP BREAST IMPLANT SCANDAL

PATIENT HARM TRIGGERING REGULATORY CHANGE

In 1965, the French plastic surgeon Henri Arion introduced the idea of implants for breast augmentation. To help support the commercial aspect of his new idea he teamed up with the butcher turned medical sales representative Jean-Claude Mas. Following Arion's death in a plane crash, Mas continued alone and in 1991 launched his own breast implant manufacturing business: Poly Implant Prothèse (PIP).

Over the following 20 years, PIP would produce some 2 million sets of breast implants and whilst initially regulatory guidelines were followed, as the business began to develop so too did the implants. Through the 90s, PIP changed the makeup of its implants from hydrogel to saline before, in 2001, Mas approved the manufacture of silicone implants using PIP's own "in house" formula. This was an industrial grade silicone that was not approved for medical use.

It was not until 2009 that concerns around the PIP silicone implants were raised. Surgeons in France were observing abnormally high rates of implant rupture, well over double the industry average. What's more, these ruptured implants appeared to cause chemical burns with localised inflammation and a profound scarring process. In 2011, the French authorities banned the use of PIP silicone implants and recommended some 30,000 French women seek removal of their implants. Mas was later arrested and sentenced to four years in prison.

The effects of the PIP scandal have been far reaching, with some 47,000 women still living with these potentially dangerous implants in the UK alone. A loophole in the regulatory framework of the time meant Mas was able to modify his previously approved implant design without seeking re-accreditation. The EU was quick to act, introducing a new Medical Devices Regulatory (MDR) framework, which now strictly governs the introduction of any new medical devices into clinical practice.

THE UK BLOOD SCANDAL

WE NEVER KNOW ALL THE RISKS TO PATIENTS

Haemophilia is an inherited condition that inhibits the normal clotting process, resulting in prolonged bleeding times and easy bruising. Throughout the 20th century, treatment for haemophiliacs was largely conservative, requiring extended hospital stays, with many whole blood transfusions to "top-up" the abnormal clotting factors.

A revolutionary new treatment brought hope to many haemophiliacs in the early 1970s. A so called "factor concentrate" was a one of blood transfusion of isolated clotting factors in far greater concentration than regular whole blood. Supplies quickly ran scarce.

The production of factor concentrate was labour intensive with as many as 60,000 blood donations mixed together to manufacture a single batch. This resulted in pharmaceutical companies sourcing often unethical new blood donors to meet demands. Prisoners, prostitutes, and intravenous drug addicts were all paid to give blood. One Canadian company even harvested blood from Russian cadavers.

All this at a time when medicine was naïve to the presence of bloodborne viruses; hepatitis C was only just being recognised and nothing was known of HIV. With pharmaceutical companies seeking higher and higher risk donors, many thousands of batches became contaminated before transfusion into NHS patients.

As a result, it is believed that through the 1970s and 80s, nearly 4,000 patients were unknowingly infected with Hepatitis C or HIV (or both), resulting in 1,246 confirmed deaths. One study published in 1986 showed that over three quarters of patients who received the novel factor concentrate went on to develop HIV. The Infected Blood Inquiry is an ongoing public statutory inquiry to examine these events. To date no one has admitted liability and no damages have been paid to the affected patients or their families.

ALDER HEY ORGAN SCANDAL

ISSUES RESULTING IN THE HUMAN TISSUE ACT 2004

Alder Hey Children's Hospital is a tertiary healthcare provider located in Liverpool. It is one of the largest and most specialised children's hospitals in the UK. Yet between 1988 and 1995 the hospital participated in the illegal removal and retention of organs from nearly a thousand children.

Accusations were made following a similar scandal at the Bristol Royal Infirmary, where the heart of an 11-month-old patient who died during open heart surgery was retained without consent in 1992. In December 1999 a formal investigation was launched at Alder Hey.

The results finally appeared in the "Redfern Report" in January of 2001. It was revealed that the pathologist at Alder Hey, Dick van Velzen, had insisted upon the "unethical and illegal stripping of every organ from every child who had had a post-mortem", even in instances where the parents had explicitly refused a full post-mortem. In addition, Alder Hey was also found to be storing 1,500 stillborn foetuses without consent.

The hospital was further criticised when it came to light that during heart surgery, children's thymus glands were being removed and given to pharmaceutical companies in return for "financial donations". The Redfern report concluded with an estimation of some 104,000 unregulated human tissue samples being stored in 210 different NHS facilities.

By 2004, Alder Hey had paid nearly £5 million in compensation to the families of victims and over 1,000 unidentified bodies (many not whole) had been released for burial. Dick van Velzen would never face criminal charges, but on 20th June 2005 he was permanently suspended from clinical practice by the GMC.

In the wake of the Alder Hey organ scandal, the Human Tissue Act was passed in 2004 to "regulate the removal, storage, use, and disposal of human bodies, organs and tissue". In particular it permits anonymous organ donation and prohibits the sale of organs. In addition, it demands that any public display of human tissue must carry a license.

BRISTOL HEART SCANDAL

A SEMINAL MOMENT IN CLINICAL GOVERNENCE

Dr Stephen Bolsin joined the Bristol Royal Infirmary (BRI) hospital in 1988 as an anaesthetist. He noticed high surgical mortality rates among paediatric patients undergoing cardiac surgery. Dr Bolsin raised these concerns to superiors in an effort to improve safety but was frustrated at the lack of action in the face of poor clinical outcomes. Consequently, he took his concerns to the media, and in doing so became a 'whistle-blower'. For this he was ostracised by colleagues, lost his job, and at a European cardiac surgeons meeting, he was described as 'the most hated anaesthetist in Europe'. He subsequently emigrated to Australia with his family and thereafter became a professor.

It has since been estimated that between 1986-1995, 170 children died at the BRI who would have survived in other NHS hospitals. The Bristol hospital Chief Executive was struck off the GMC medical register in 1997 for professional misconduct as part of the fall out. In 1998, an investigation was set up that resulted in the Kennedy report which found that systemic, cultural failings contributed to the poor safety record at Bristol.

Clinical governance is an umbrella term used to describe the systematic approach to maintaining and improving the quality of patient care. Since the Bristol heart scandal, it has become crucial to be able to demonstrate that the medical profession is protecting patients from unacceptable care. One of the pillars of clinical governance is audit of care and outcomes against specific criteria in order to undertake targeted quality improvement initiatives. This is a crucial part of delivery of care, and involvement in this is a requirement of all doctors.

> There are 7 pillars of clinical governance: clinical effectiveness and research; audit; risk management and minimisation; education and training; patient and public involvement in discussions; appropriate use of information and IT; appropriate staffing and staff management.

THE MMR VACCINE AND AUTISM

BAD SCIENCE

In 1998, Andrew Wakefield published an article in the Lancet documenting a case series linking the measles, mumps, and rubella (MMR) vaccine to the development of autism in later life. The MMR vaccine at the time, as it still is now, was part of the national routine neonatal immunisation schedule and was therefore being offered to every child in the UK. A media frenzy ensued and MMR vaccination rates began to fall dramatically.

Huge epidemiological studies followed almost immediately, drawing on national databases containing records for thousands of patients. A stark contrast to Wakefield's un-controlled case report of just 12 patients. Results of these larger studies quickly refuted and dismissed Wakefield's claims as false. Soon after the authors published a retraction withdrawing their previous conclusions but it was too late, the damage was done, and anti-vaccination movements were growing. MMR uptake continued to fall.

Over the following decade Wakefield's work was interrogated and revealed, shockingly, that his invalid conclusions went beyond simply incorrect scientific acumen, but were in fact blatantly fraudulent. The 12 patients included in Wakefield's study were not randomly selected, they were hand-picked, and the details from their medical care were carefully selected or even falsified to construct an argument for the story Wakefield wanted to tell. It soon came to light that Wakefield was receiving payments from anti-vaccination lawyers so it is likely all of this was done for financial gain.

Whilst Wakefield has now been thoroughly discredited (and even struck of the medical register), the effects of what was one of the biggest medical frauds in history are still apparent. MMR vaccination rates have never fully recovered and measles outbreaks in 2008, 2009, and 2013 have all been attributed to the doubt and fear cast by Wakefield's falsified conclusions.

This saga serves as a constant reminder that scientific research should remain unbiased and impartial. Researchers that publish their work have an ethical responsibility to maintain the highest levels of scientific rigour and avoid errors or deceit that may ultimately lead to patient harm.

THERALIZUMAB DRUG TRIAL

A CATASTROPHIC DRUG TRIAL THAT SPARKED REFORM

In 2006, a new drug that modulated the immune system was developed. This drug was TGN1412 and it was a monoclonal antibody that bound to the human CD28 receptor found on T cells. When a CD28 receptor is bound to, the T cell it is found on is activated. In rodent models it was shown that the drug preferentially activated a class of T cells called regulatory T cells that suppress the immune response. As such the drug was intended to treat Rheumatoid arthritis, a disease where the body's immune system is persistently activated, and targets tissue in joints and other organs (autoimmunity).

TGN1412 passed all safety tests that precede clinical trials, and in 2006, six healthy humans were part of the first phase-I clinical trials. All six developed systemic inflammatory responses and became critically ill. Two of the six required intensive organ support for over a week. One man developed a swollen head, leading to the trial being dubbed the 'Elephant man trial'.

An investigation concluded that it was unforeseen biological effects not predicated by pre-clinical trials that caused the serious reactions. This was due to mis-interpretation of the results of primate studies, insufficient *in-vitro* human studies, and a miscalculation in the starting dose of the drug. This impact of unforeseen effects was compounded by all six recipients being administered the drug within ten minutes of each other, thus allowing no time for the observation of possible unexpected side effects.

Following this trial, changes to European guidelines were put in place to identify and mitigate risk in phase I trials of biologic drugs (drugs produced from, or containing components of living organisms such as antibodies). A number of regulatory and advisory checks were put in place concerning the close scrutiny of preclinical analyses. Guidelines have been put in place about the initial drug administration in humans; this should be done over several hours with frequent evaluation of participants, and should occur at sites with immediate access to treatment.

SWINE FLU PANDEMIC

THE 2009 H1N1 SWINE INFLUENZA PANDEMIC

Flu, also known as Influenza, is a respiratory illness caused by the influenza virus. There are four types of influenza virus: A, B, C and D. These are distinguished based on differences in internal proteins. Types A, B, and C can all infect humans. Types A and B are responsible for the vast majority of seasonal epidemics (widespread winter flu), however whilst Influenza B viruses circulate almost exclusively in humans, Influenza A viruses infect humans and other animals such as pigs and birds. Therefore, type A viruses are of most significance to public health as they can potentially cause pandemics.

Subtypes of each type of virus are distinguished from each other by the proteins they express on their surface. Influenza A viruses are distinguished by containing two proteins called Hemagglutinin (HA) and Neuraminidase (NA). Being external proteins, HA and NA determine what the virus binds to, and the extent of the infected animal's immune reaction.

There are 18 known HA subtypes (H1 through H18) and 11 known NA subtypes (N1 through N11). Each virus will have one type of each, and many different combinations of these HA and NA proteins are possible. Currently H1N1 and H3N2 are the main Influenza A viruses circulating in humans.

Swine flu was the unofficial name given to the H1N1 strain that was responsible for the 2009-10 flu pandemic. At the time, this was a strain that was found in large numbers of pigs but had not been transmitted to humans any more than a handful of times in 50 years; each time only causing a few infections. Consequently, very few humans had any immunity to this strain from previous exposure, and it was not vaccinated against. This led to concern that a virulent new flu strain would spread through populations with ease.

Since 2009, the same H1N1 strain has become endemic in humans around the world and is now considered a normal seasonal flu strain that is vaccinated against.

NOVICHOK AGENTS

NERVE AGENTS THAT POISONED THE SKRIPAL'S IN SALISBURY, UK

Nerve agents are chemicals that target the nervous system. Novichok agents are a sub-type of nerve agents that were designed in Russia during the Cold War as chemical weapons. In March 2018, two Russians, Sergei and Yulia Skripal, were poisoned with Novichok in Salisbury. Subsequently, a number of people in the Salisbury area have been affected to some degree by Novichok, notably one woman who died after coming into contact with the discarded container of Novichok.

Nerve agents cause morbidity and often death via a 'cholinergic crisis'. They inhibit the enzyme acetylcholinesterase (AChE), which normally acts to reduce the amount of acetylcholine (ACh) in synapses in the body, in particular at the junction between nerves and muscles (the neuromuscular junction). Muscles normally respond to ACh by contracting, but an excessive build-up of ACh following inhibition of AChE results in muscles, including the crucial muscles that drive respiration, become overwhelmed with ACh and instead respond by becoming flaccid. This can be deadly if the diaphragm is affected. Other symptoms of exposure to nerve agents are stimulation of salivary glands, urination, defecation, and constriction of pupils.

Treatment is a dual therapy of an anticholinergic drug such as atropine (to mitigate the action of all the excess ACh in synapses by blocking the ACh receptor) and an oxime drug (to re-activate the AChE enzymes to start to break down the ACh again).

Some common pesticides and insecticides are made of organophosphate compounds, which, like nerve agents, inhibit AChE. Insecticide poisoning is a form of suicide and something medical professionals must be aware of.

EBOLA

A SEVERE DISEASE CAUSED BY EBOLA VIRUS

Ebola, also known as Ebola virus disease (EVD) is a severe disease caused by Ebola virus, which infects humans, primates, and bats.

The disease occurs mainly in Sub-Saharan Africa. Since first being identified in 1976, the largest outbreak was between 2013 and 2016 in west Africa where there were around 29,000 cases and 11,000 deaths.

Ebola is a viral haemorrhagic fever that kills around 50% of those infected. Symptoms of Ebola start as a fever, and can progress to internal and external haemorrhage (bleeding). The virus spreads with direct contact of body fluids such as blood, faeces, and vomit.

Once a patient has recovered from Ebola, the virus is cleared from the blood, saliva, and most organs. However, there is evidence that it can remain in the eye, the central nervous system and, in men, in the testes and semen for some time. These sites are known as 'immune-privileged sites' as foreign antibodies that access them do not tend to trigger an immune response.

It is believed that Ebola is a zoonotic pathogen and whilst the natural reservoir for Ebola has not been confirmed, bats are the most likely candidate. They carry the virus without getting unwell, unlike humans and primates.

> Health-care workers treated those with Ebola are at greatest risk of infection, especially if there is a lack of personal protective equipment. In December 2014, a British nurse who had worked with Ebola patients in Sierra Leone was diagnosed with Ebola in Glasgow. Following this she was transferred to the Royal Free in London for specialist high-level isolation care. She was discharge in January 2015, after being declared free of the virus. In late 2015, she was re-admitted an Ebola virus was found in her cerebrospinal fluid, where it had remained. She was treated for meningitis caused by Ebola virus but subsequently made a full recovery.

SEVERE ACUTE RESPIRATORY SYNDROME CORONAVIRUS 2

VIROLOGY OF SARS-COV-2

Severe acute respiratory syndrome–related coronavirus (SARSr-CoV) is a species of virus (of the family *Coronaviridae* and genus *Betacoronavirus*) containing different strains of viruses that are related to the SARS-CoV-1 virus responsible for the 2002-2004 outbreak of severe acute respiratory syndrome (SARS). There are many known strains of SARSr-CoV that were found during research into the natural reservoir of SARS-CoV-1, and although many do not infect humans, in 2016, the species was identified as a likely cause of future epidemic. Aside from SARS-CoV-1 the only other strain of SARSr-CoV to have caused an outbreak in humans is SARS-COV-2, the virus that caused coronavirus-2019 disease (COVID-19).

The original source of SARS-CoV-2 transmission to humans is unclear. Analysis of viral genetic data can indicate whether viruses are epidemiologically linked. Analysis of SARS-CoV-2 from early patients showed a high degree of relation, consistent with a common ancestor in late 2019.

There are thousands of variants of SARS-CoV-2, each with a genetic mutation causing an amino acid change. The World Health Organisation declares some variants as 'variants of concern' or 'variants under investigation' when the amino acid change confers a selection advantage to the virus, such as increased transmissibility.

> Following the 2002-2004 SARS outbreak caused by the SARS-CoV-1 virus, there was an effort to search for similar viruses with the potential to infect humans. Virologists took to searching animal populations and sequencing the genomes of viruses they found. A large number of SARS-related coronaviruses (SARSr-CoV) were detected in horseshoe bats around Asia, and there were a number of papers written warning of the need to prepare for future emergence of SARS-like diseases.

COVID-19

CORONAVIRUS-2019 DISEASE (COVID-19)

Coronavirus-2019 disease (COVID-19) is an infectious disease caused by the SARS-CoV-2 virus.

The first confirmed human cases of infection with the severe acute respiratory syndrome coronavirus 2 (SARS-CoV-2) were in Wuhan, China. This virus is responsible for causing COVID-19 (coronavirus disease 2019), the respiratory illness that has since driven the COVID-19 pandemic.

A large number of people infected with SARS-COV-2 remain asymptomatic. If symptomatic, COVID-19 presents itself in patients in a heterogenous manner but those most unwell with the disease will have multi-system involvement. This classically involves difficulty breathing caused by respiratory failure but also coagulation abnormalities and microvascular blood vessel damage affecting the brain and kidneys. People who are unwell with COVID-19 will have raised levels of blood pro-inflammatory markers, and a 'cytokine storm' causing extreme systemic inflammation can be a complication.

Treatments for COVID-19 are developing. The first major breakthrough in management was made by the RECOVERY clinical trial in the UK, which showed that Dexamethasone (a cheap and ubiquitous corticosteroid) reduces mortality rates by one third in those requiring supplemental oxygen.

Due to the mortality rate of COVID-19, countries around the world attempted to put in place significant public health efforts to stop the spread of SARS-COV-2. A number of vaccines were developed, and countries instigated lock-downs and mandatory wearing of face masks.

> The RECOVERY trial is a UK based trial undertaken within the NHS. This is a large scale randomised trial which enrols those who have been hospitalised with COVID-19 and assigns them to a treatment arm. The trial was set up very quickly following the pandemic, and has become a 'poster-child' for the speed with which ethical approval and trial organisation can work. It is hoped that this will be replicated in clinical trials in fields other than COVID-19.

www.ingramcontent.com/pod-product-compliance
Lightning Source LLC
Chambersburg PA
CBHW070118230526
45472CB00004B/1322